NEUROSCIENCE NURSING
A Nursing Diagnosis
Approach

NEUROSCIENCE NURSING
A Nursing Diagnosis Approach

MARILYNN MITCHELL,
R.N., M.S.N., C.N.R.N.

Head Nurse
Neuroscience Intensive Care Unit
    and Rehabilitation Unit
Denver General Hospital
Denver, Colorado

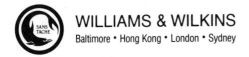

WILLIAMS & WILKINS
Baltimore • Hong Kong • London • Sydney

Editor: Margo C. Neal
Associate Editor: Marjorie Kidd Keating
Copy Editor: Barbara Werner
Design: Dan Pfisterer
Illustration Planning: Lorraine Wrzosek
Production: Anne G. Seitz

Copyright © 1989
Williams & Wilkins
428 East Preston Street
Baltimore, Maryland 21202, USA

Accurate indications, adverse reactions, and dosage schedules for
drugs are provided in this book, but it is possible that they may
change. The reader is urged to review the package information data of
the manufacturers of the medications mentioned.

Printed in the United States of America

Library of Congress Cataloging-in-Publication Data
Neuroscience nursing.
    Includes index.
    1. Neurological nursing. I. Mitchell, Marilynn
[DNLM: 1. Nervous System Diseases—nursing. 2. Nursing
Assessment. WY 160 N49465]
RC350.5.N488   1989   610.73'68   88-20452
ISBN 0-683-06099-6

                                        88 89 90 91 92
                                    1 2 3 4 5 6 7 8 9 10

FOREWORD

Nothing gives me greater satisfaction than seeing an expert practitioner translate that very special blend of science and art that is so integral a part of master practice into a written work. I firmly believe that few things are more powerful in terms of influencing the nursing practice of others than a well-written book. In *Neuroscience Nursing: A Nursing Diagnosis Approach*, the author has brought years of clinical experience and melded that experience into a practical and realistic text.

Nurses today are forced to cope with a multitude of serious issues that impinge on nursing practice. Consider the nursing shortage, runaway technology, sicker and sicker patients, concern for legalities, diagnosis-related groups, and the demands for documentation of care, to name just a few. As a result, there is a realistic concern about compromised patient outcomes, and achieving the goal of quality care for patients has become more elusive. Application of nursing diagnoses holds the promise of assisting us in the challenges of facing these dilemmas. Yet, the concept of nursing diagnosis has had its problems with acceptance. What Marilynn Mitchell does is operationalize this concept where it really counts—at the bedside. Her application of nursing diagnoses is a unique feature of the book and hopefully will encourage further utilization in the clinical setting.

Rarely are health problems as devastating as those encountered in the neuroscience arena. At the same time, few areas in nursing seem to intimidate practitioners more than dysfunctions of the nervous system. Caring for these patients requires an exceptional blend of compassion and intellectual reasoning. One without the other robs the patient of the essence of professional nursing. A resource that can translate seemingly difficult concepts into manageable ones and provide a framework for the day-to-day nursing care of patients with these disorders is indeed welcome.

Carolyn M. Hudak, R.N., Ph.D
Denver, Colorado

PREFACE

Accurate nursing assessments and quick interventions are critical in neuroscience nursing, perhaps more so than in other fields of nursing. The reason for this is that nursing actions may actually determine patient outcome. How quickly a nurse recognizes the significance of a change may determine the degree of neurologic injury and the permanent deficit that will be with the patient for the remainder of his or her life.

There is a specific body of neuroscience knowledge that nurses caring for neurologically injured patients need to know. There are specific assessment skills necessary to be able to recognize a subtle change in neurologic status and its significance.

Over the years, student nurses and nurses new to neuroscience nursing have questioned the "why" of patient behavior and the "why" of clinical signs as related to neuroanatomy. This book is an attempt to relate the pathophysiology to the clinical signs and the nursing intervention (in nursing diagnosis format) needed.

ACKNOWLEDGMENTS

I would like to acknowledge the nursing administration and staff nurses of the neurointensive care, intermediate care, and rehabilitation units at Denver General Hospital for allowing me the opportunity to function as Head Nurse of those units and gain and share my knowledge about neuroscience nursing.

CONTENTS

Section 1

NEUROSCIENCE
HEALTH PROBLEMS

Section 2

NEUROSCIENCE
NURSING

INTRODUCTION

This book is meant to be a practical resource for nurses in neurointensive care units, emergency departments, neuro-step-down units, medical-surgical units, and rehabilitation units; for nursing students studying neuroscience; and for faculty.

The pathophysiology is related to clinical signs and symptoms. The nursing intervention is written in nursing diagnosis format. The nursing diagnoses are cross-referenced so they may be applicable to patients with several neurologic disorders or injuries. Nursing care plans should be easily extracted based on the nursing diagnoses and the intervention listed.

SECTION 1

NEUROSCIENCE HEALTH PROBLEMS

Neuroscience Assessment

I. BEDSIDE ASSESSMENT

Much of the assessment we perform in a neuro check on a hospitalized patient is subjective. The data cannot be quantified like the data we gather with a stethoscope in measuring blood pressure, for instance. It takes a trained assessor to evaluate neurological parameters. As bedside nurses, we must be able to perform in this role of assessor.

Level of Consciousness

The single most important observation that can be made of a neurologically injured patient is the level of consciousness. Clinically, this is the parameter that will change the earliest to indicate an improvement or deterioration in the patient's condition. Consciousness is a dynamic state, changing with time. It is an awareness of oneself and the environment. It is dependent upon two primary areas in the brain, the reticular activation system (RAS) and the cortex. Both areas must be intact for normal consciousness. (Fig. 1.1)

The RAS in the brainstem receives input from the environment such as proprioception and pressure information. This information is transmitted to the cortex, resulting in arousal. Injury to the RAS or cortex results in a depression in level of consciousness. Increased intracranial pressure against the RAS fibers also can impede stimulation to the cortex.

A meaningful assessment and communication of that assessment has been difficult to achieve. Fairly recently, however, since the Glasgow Coma Scale has come into more universal use, terms such as "stuporous," "semicomatose," "delirious," and "comatose," which may have very different meanings to different examiners, are not being used so much. The universal way to describe level of consciousness is with the Glasgow Coma Scale, and terms have the same meaning to all observers.

The scale evaluates three parameters: eye opening, verbal response, and

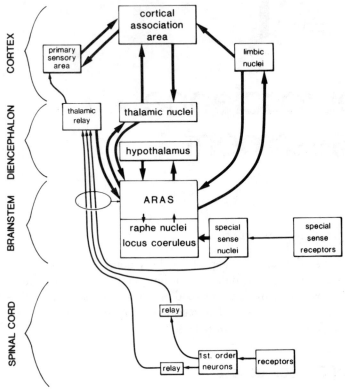

Figure 1.1. Schematic diagram of arousal pathways. ARAS is the Ascending Reticular Activating System. (Reproduced with permission from Snyder M: *A Guide to Neurological and Neurosurgical Nursing.* New York, Wiley & Sons 1983, p 101.)

motor response. The patient is given a score for the best response he can achieve. The rating scale is shown in Table 1.1.

The scores range from 3 to 15. A score of 7 or less is defined as coma. Paramedics can assign a coma score to a patient in the field. This can be communicated to the Emergency Department, and then to the Intensive Care Unit. It is helpful to a nurse, even without a detailed report about the patient, to know the coma score. A score of 12 tells the nurse the patient is primarily being admitted for observation. A score of 5 tells the nurse the patient will be unresponsive to all but painful stimuli, will likely be intubated and have other lines, such as a nasogastric tube and arterial line, and will require a great deal of nursing care.

Other aspects of a mental status exam can be assessed at the bedside, often simply by conversing with the patient. Orientation can be ascertained by asking the patient for specific information, such as the name of the presi-

Table 1.1.
Rating Scale

Eye Opening	
Nil	= 1
To pain	= 2
To speech	= 3
Spontaneous	= 4

Best Verbal Response	
Nil	= 1
Incomprehensible sounds	= 2
Inappropriate words	= 3
Confused conversation	= 4
Oriented	= 5

Best Motor Response	
Flaccid	= 1
Extension	= 2
Abnormal flexion	= 3
Flexor withdrawal	= 4
Localized to pain	= 5
Obeys commands	= 6

dent or today's date. Disorientation to place and person implies a more serious cerebral disorder than does disorientation to time.

Recent memory can be checked by asking the patient what he ate for his last meal. Remote memory can be tested by having the patient recall his birthdate or a special time or place of an event. Remote memory tends to survive acquired disease.

Abstract reasoning can be tested by asking the patient to interpret a proverb, or asking the patient how two things are alike, such as an apple and an orange. Ability to calculate may be checked with serial sevens (ask the patient to count backward from 100, subtracting seven each time).

Speech and language may also be noted at the bedside. A defect in articulation, enunciation, and rhythm of speech (dysarthria) would be noticeable. Dysphonia, a disorder of vocalization with abnormal production of sounds from the larynx, may be present. Dysphasia is an inability to use and understand spoken or written language. Nonfluent dysphasia describes a patient who produces few or no words. He is unable to respond verbally, although his comprehension may be good. Fluent dysphasia involves a normal amount of words produced, but the content is confused. Words with no meaning may be produced, or words may be used incorrectly in a sentence.

Pupil Check

Pupils are checked for size, shape, reaction to light, and symmetry. Pupils are normally round and equal. Their size may vary from about 2 to 6 mm in diameter, depending greatly on the environmental light.

Unequal pupils do not necessarily mean the patient has increased intracranial pressure. Direct orbital trauma, drugs, eye drops, or an eye prosthesis could all account for an inequality. The more depressed the level of consciousness, the more likely that a unilateral fixed and dilated pupil represents herniation of brain structures secondary to increased intracranial pressure.

The third cranial nerves control the pupils' ability to constrict. They are located along the transtentorial notch. When the brain becomes edematous from a supratentorial injury, pressure builds because the skull cannot expand. The increasing pressure pushes on the brain, which also compresses the third cranial nerve. The pupil on the same side as the lesion or pressure will dilate and become nonreactive to light.

Pupils should be checked for direct light reaction and also for consensual light response. When light is shone directly in one eye, the pupil should constrict. This is the direct light reflex. When there is constriction of the non-stimulated eye, this is the consensual light reflex. The crossing of some fibers in the optic chiasm accounts for consensual reflex. A parasympathetic lesion or third cranial nerve lesion is often suspected if a pupil is sluggish to react to direct light and there is no consensual response.

Accommodation cannot be checked in unconscious patients. This refers to the refractory power of the lens. It involves voluntary focus on a nearby or faraway object.

Pupil changes are often late signs of increased intracranial pressure or of herniation. The observation of a patient's deteriorating condition should be made when the level of consciousness changes. Once pupil changes have occurred, it may be too late to save the patient.

Pupils do not always become large, dilated and nonreactive to light when the patient is getting into trouble. Patients with subarachnoid hemorrhages may have a central herniation and initially small reactive pupils. So, it is a change from the individual's baseline that we look for.

Vital Signs

Changes in vital signs are another usually late indication of neurological deterioration. The typical initial cardiovascular response to increasing intracranial pressure (ICP) is an increase in mean arterial pressure and bradycardia.

The medulla in the brainstem has a major role in regulating blood vessel diameter (BP). When there is an increase in ICP, pressure is placed on the medulla, and it becomes hypoxic. This results in arterial hypertension, which is a mechanism the body uses to try to increase the cerebral perfusion so that the brain can get more oxygen. Bradycardia is due to pressure on the vasomotor center, increasing transmission of parasympathetic impulses, thus slowing heart rate.

The mechanism of increasing the mean arterial pressure requires an intact medulla. Cardiovascular changes do not take place when the medulla is destroyed. Prolonged compression of the medulla paralyzes the medullary centers. This results in hypotension, tachycardia and, eventually, respiratory arrest.

The Cushing response (widening pulse pressure and bradycardia) is a normal cardiovascular change when the medulla is intact, and it is clinically significant when it occurs. It signals threatening decompensation in the balance of pressure in the head. Unfortunately this typical response is not always present, even when the ICP has elevated rapidly.

Respiratory changes may occur, depending on the level of brain injury. On a neuroanatomical basis from higher to lower areas in the brain, breathing patterns usually seen are: Cheyne-Stokes, central neurogenic hyperventilation, apneustic breathing, cluster breathing, and ataxic or Biot's respirations.

Temperature changes may or may not be seen clinically. A factor in temperature changes is the amount of edema or pressure in the hypothalamic region of the brain. Hyperthermia is damaging to a patient with increased intracranial pressure, because it increases the metabolic demands of the brain.

Motor Response

The motor assessment done in a routine bedside neuro check should include observation for symmetry of extremities. Look at limb position. In a comatose patient there is usually symmetrical positioning. If the extremities are not positioned symmetrically, it could be a focal sign, that is, there is a brain lesion on one side.

Look at the tone of the extremities. They are usually flaccid in comatose patients. Hypoxia can often cause an increase in tone, and that is acceptable unless it is asymmetrical.

Extremity strength should be tested. Hand grasping is a gross test of hand strength. To test the strength in the upper extremity, the patient should be asked to hold both arms outstretched in front of his body, palms up, fingers spread, and eyes closed. A gradual drift and pronation of an arm is a reliable sign of paresis of that extremity.

To test lower extremity strength, the patient should be asked to raise his legs up off the bed. Having a patient push against the nurse's hand on the sole of the patient's foot tests Achilles tendon strength, but does not fully test the motor strength in the leg.

In an unconscious patient, both arms can be lifted and released simultaneously. If one arm falls more rapidly and in a flail-like manner, it could be paralyzed or have a weakness. To test leg strength in a comatose patient, the nurse can flex the patient's legs so that both heels are on the bed. Once the legs are released, they should hold the position for a few moments, then gradually return to the pretesting position. A weak or paralyzed leg will often slump to a position of extension with outward rotation of the hip.

There are two types of abnormal body positioning seen in neurologically impaired patients: decorticate (flexion) and decerebrate (extension) positions. The lower extremities are basically the same in both positions, they are stiffly extended with plantar flexion. Decorticate positioning involves a flexion of the arms at the elbows and wrists, and adduction at the shoulders. In decerebrate posturing, the arms are stiffly extended, adducted, and hyperpronated, and the wrists and fingers flexed.

Decorticate posturing often indicates a lesion in a cerebral hemisphere. Decerebrate posturing indicates a brainstem injury. A patient may fluctuate between these two types of motor responses, due to variation in the blood supply to the involved area of the brain.

Abnormal Reflexes

Presence of some abnormal reflexes may be seen in neurologically injured patients. Determination of reflex eye movements is the most useful bedside test of the functional integrity of the brainstem in an unconscious patient. The oculovestibular reflex (Doll's eyes phenomenon or proprioceptive head turning) may be tested at the bedside. To test for the reflex, hold the unconscious patient's eyelids open. Then quickly turn his head first to one side and then the other. When the reflex is present, the patient's eyes will move to the opposite direction from the side to which the head was turned. When there is severe brainstem involvement, the Doll's eyes reflex disappears. Instead, only one eye may move, or both may not move at all.

Normally the reflex is present to allow a person to voluntarily fix his vision on a point while his body is moving. If this reflex is not present, one of three things may be happening. The brainstem may be destroyed, the person is faking coma, or the person is in a metabolic or toxic coma (this reflex disappears late in the course of metabolic encephalopathy).

Since cervical spine injury must be ruled out before rotating the head, and because Doll's eyes is a weaker reflex than caloric stimulation oculovestibular or calorics is often a preferred test. If Doll's eyes are positive, there is no need to do calorics.

To test for the oculovestibular reflex (calorics), the head of the bed is elevated 30° to bring the lateral semicircular canal into a vertical position, and 20–50 cc of ice water is irrigated against the tympanic membrane.

In a normal, awake patient, the response is nystagmus that is regular, rhythmic, and lasts 2 to 3 minutes. There is little excursion of the eye from midline. As consciousness is lost from brain injury, the fast component progressively disappears and the slow component carries the eyes tonically toward the irrigated ear.

Five minutes should elapse before performing the caloric test in the opposite ear. Response in patients with brainstem injuries may be downward deviation of both eyes or one eye, dysconjugate eye movements, or no response at all.

This cold caloric test evaluates lateral eye movements. To test vertical eye movements, one can irrigate both auditory canals simultaneously with ice water. In a comatose patient with an intact brainstem, the eyes deviate downward. To produce upward gaze, either irrigate both canals with warm water simultaneously or position the head 60 degrees below the horizontal and use ice water.

Deep tendon reflexes (DTR's) may be part of the bedside assessment. Bicep, knee jerk, and brachial radialis reflexes can be a quick and reliable check, without doing a complete DTR check. In the unconscious patient, unilateral hyperreflexes along with pathological reflexes indicate hemiparesis.

Muscle response to reflex testing is graded from 0 to 4. Grade 0 indicates the reflex is absent. Grade 1 indicates it is diminished. Grade 2 is a normal reflex. Grade 3 is a reflex brisker than normal. Grade 4 is a hyperactive reflex (clonus).

Babinski reflex should also be part of the motor exam. The lateral aspect of the sole of the foot is stroked with a blunt point. The normal response in adults is flexion of the toes (downward). Abnormal response to the stroking is when the great toe dorsiflexes (pulls upward) and the other toes fan downward. This response is a Babinski. It is present or not present (not positive or negative). When it is present it may indicate an upper motor neuron lesion or paralysis.

Sensory Evaluation

The patient should be awake in order to give subjective interpretation of sensory stimuli for a full sensory examination. The sensory assessment should include response to pain, temperature, light touch and pressure, discriminative touch, proprioception, and vibration. As in the motor examination, symmetry should be noted. The stimuli should be scattered over the patient's body in order to cover most dermatomes and major peripheral nerves.

Superficial pain may be tested by using a safety pin and having the patient describe the sensation as sharp or dull, alternating the use of the sharp and blunt ends of the pin. If pain sensation is normal, there may be no need to test the patient for temperature sensation.

Light touch can be evaluated by touching the patient with a wisp of cotton and having him describe where the touch was. A vibrating tuning fork over a distal interphalangeal joint of a finger and the great toe tests vibration sensation.

Two-point discrimination tests discriminative sensation. The patient closes his eyes and is touched on two parts of the body simultaneously and is asked to identify where the touching occurred. Point localization may also be helpful. The patient is touched while his eyes are closed and then is asked to open his eyes and point to the area touched.

Deep pain may be tested for in unconscious patients. This may be done by squeezing the trapezius or the Achilles tendon. Sternal pressure with the examiner's knuckles may be a strong pain stimulus, but the patient may develop bruising over the area. Supraorbital pressure is also a painful stimulus. Pressure to the tip of the fingernail or toenail, such as with a pencil, may also elicit a painful response.

The Romberg test is used to test for position sense in the legs and trunk. Joint motion and position are part of the test for proprioception. This may be done by having the patient close his eyes as the examiner moves the distal phalanx of one of the fingers upward or downward and asking the patient to describe the direction of movement.

It is not practical to try to examine all areas of the body for sensory function. A history of numbness or tingling or the feeling of pins and needles may guide the examiner to specific areas of the body. The perimeter of an involved area should be determined to try to localize the possible area of a lesion causing the sensory deficit.

Cranial Nerves

Cranial nerves may or may not be able to be assessed at the bedside, depending upon the amount of cooperation the patient can give the examiner, and the patient's level of consciousness. Table 1.2 indicates the function of the cranial nerves and how they may be tested.

In summary, any bedside neuro check should include an assessment of level of consciousness, pupil check, vital signs, motor and sensory responses, abnormal reflexes, and possibly cranial nerves. Interpretation of the observations we make at the bedside helps us to decide what action, if any, needs to be taken. Some neurological changes are very subtle, so it is vital to establish an accurate initial neurological baseline.

II. HISTORY

A neurologic history should be a part of any general medical workup, because many disorders of other body systems present with neurologic complaints. Hypertension, cirrhosis, and diabetes mellitus are several disorders with possible neurologic involvement. Neurologic signs may also be seen as a result of drugs being taken for a nonneurologic problem.

A patient with a neurologic problem may or may not be able to give a reliable and accurate history. Altered mental status, inaccurate perception of the

Table 1.2.
Cranial Nerve Functions and Tests

Cranial Nerve	Function	Test
I Olfactory	Smell	Ask patient to identify familiar odors.
II Optic	Visual fields and acuity	Determine visual fields by confrontation. Use Snellen chart to assess acuity of vision.
III Oculomotor	Pupillary constriction; accommodation; movement of eye nasally, down and in, and up and lateral; eyelid opening	Have patient follow examiner's finger in all directions while holding the head straight ahead. Check for ptosis of eyelids.
IV Trochlear	Downward and outward movement of eye	Have patient move eye in and down.
V Trigeminal	Muscles of mastication	Ask patient to clench his teeth. Test for corneal reflex. Have patient identify sharp and dull sensation over forehead and cheek and jaw.
VI Abducens	Lateral eye movements	Have patient move eyes laterally.
VII Facial	Eyelid closing; movement of muscles of face and scalp, taste sensation on anterior ⅔ of tongue	Have patient raise eyebrows, frown, close eyes tightly, show his teeth, smile, puff out checks. Have patient identify salt and sugar on anterior part of tongue.
VIII Acoustic	Cochlear: hearing	Test for air and bone conduction. Test if patient hears ticking watch.
	Vestibular: equilibrium	Do Romberg test

(continued)

Table 1.2. (*Continued*)

Cranial Nerve	Function	Test
IX Glossopharyngeal	Taste sensation on posterior half of tongue. Pain, touch, temperature sensation of throat and pharynx. Controls muscles of pharynx	Test for gag reflex, swallowing reflex, and phonation. Check if uvula stays midline when saying "ah."
X Vagus	Sensation of larynx, trachea, esophagus, lungs. Causes bradycardia and contracts bronchial muscles. Controls muscles of pharynx and larynx.	Test together with glossopharyngeal nerve.
XI Spinal Accessory	Controls neck and shoulder muscles	Ask patient to shrug shoulders and turn his head to each side against examiner's hand.
XII Hypoglossal	Movement of tongue	Ask patient to stick out tongue. Check for tremors, asymmetry, deviation, or atrophy.

problem, or dysphasia may all hinder the patient from giving an accurate history. Family or a caregiver may be able to give a more reliable history, or at least confirm the history a patient gives.

Chief complaints often described by patients with disorders of the nervous system include:

—Headache,
—Mental status change such as confusion,
—Vertigo and loss of balance,
—Change in motor strength or coordination,
—Pain,
—Sensory disturbances such as paresthesia,
—Seizures,
—Tinnitus or loss of hearing,
—Disturbance of memory or thinking,
—Difficulty with speech or with swallowing.

The chronology of events or onset of symptoms should be determined. Date and mode of onset and duration of each sympton should be investigated. Activities and treatments which aggravate or alleviate the symptom(s) should be explored.

Neurologic complaints may be vague in nature, and some patients may fail to describe a common symptom, thinking it unimportant to relate. The examiner should ask about the following complaints if not described by the patient:

—Headache,
—Dizziness,
—Visual disturbances,
—Bladder dysfunction,
—Weakness.

Family history should be obtained as it relates to the chief complaint or chronic illnesses. The patient's social, economic, and cultural status may be important in understanding the patient's response to the chief complaint and how it is interpreted by the patient.

III. DIAGNOSTIC TESTS

There are many diagnostic tests which may be helpful in assessing a patient for a neurologic problem.

CT (computed tomography) is one of the most helpful radiological exams available today. It is painless and noninvasive. A computer analysis of tissue density provides a quick printout which can be interpreted and care then provided to head trauma victims without delay.

Patients may or may not be injected with contrast media. The advantage to a CT scan with contrast is that the cerebral vasculature is more distinct.

Indications for a CT scan may be head trauma where the physician is looking for a mass, possible hydrocephalus, atrophy, infarction, congenital defects, and to monitor cerebral swelling. Abscesses, infarctions, and aneurysms, as well as some inner ear problems may be defined on CT scan.

Cerebral angiography is an invasive procedure in which radiopaque dye is injected into the cerebral circulation and x-rays monitor the dye's progress through the vasculature. This procedure is used most often to clarify anatomic information for surgery and to evaluate vascular disorders such as aneurysms and arteriovenous malformations. Displacement of vessels can be seen, which may occur with a brain tumor, hydrocephalus, or a blood clot.

Digital subtraction angiography (DSA) is a newer type of computerized fluoroscopy which is used to visualize carotid and cerebral vessels. One scan is made and then, after the dye is injected intravenously, a second scan is made. The first image is subtracted from the second, thus heightening visualization.

Nursing Intervention with a Patient Having a CT Scan
1. Explain that his head will be immobilized and the patient must remain still. He will be asked to lie on a flat hard table.
2. Bobby pins should be removed from hair before procedure.
3. If contrast is to be used, ask the patient about allergies, especially to iodine-based dyes.
4. The patient will feel a warm flush and a metallic taste in the mouth as contrast is given. Other symptoms may be tachycardia, tachypnea, nausea, and restlessness.
5. Expect the patient to diurese after CT scan if contrast was used. Urine specific gravity may be abnormally high for up to 12 hours postprocedure. Monitoring of urine output in patients with renal problems is recommended postprocedure, to assure that the patient does not develop renal failure.
6. Contrast dye is a hypertonic solution, so it acts much as Mannitol does on cerebral edema. It may reduce the edema temporarily, and the patient may appear neurologically improved. Several hours postprocedure, however, the cerebral swelling may reappear, and the patient may rapidly deteriorate if not closely monitored.

Nursing Intervention with a Patient Having an Angiogram
1. Ask patient about allergies, especially to iodine-based dyes.
2. Tell patient to expect a flushed feeling as dye is injected, and that local anesthesia will be used at the catheter site.
3. Monitor patient during procedure and afterwards for signs of stroke (a vessel plaque may become dislodged). This includes dysphasia, hemiparesis or hemiplegia, and a change in level of consciousness.
4. Explain to patient what is going on during the procedure, to help in getting his cooperation.
5. Watch for hematoma formation or bleeding at cannulation site postprocedure. A pressure dressing may be necessary.
6. Check pulses distal to cannulation site frequently after angio.
7. The extremity used for cannulation should remain immobile several hours after procedure.
8. If subclavian approach was used, watch for signs of pneumothorax.
9. Expect patient to diurese after procedure. Urine specific gravity may be abnormally high for up to 12 hours postprocedure. Monitoring of urine output in patients with renal problems is recommended to assure the patient does not develop renal failure.

A *brain scan* involves injecting a radioisotope intravenously. Films of the isotope uptake by different areas of the brain are produced. Focal uptake may indicate hemorrhage, tumor, abscess, or infarction. The scan may not reveal specifically what the lesion is, but only that there is an abnormality. There is usually more uptake in areas where the blood brain barrier has been disturbed, in areas of cerebral infarction, and in areas of contusion.

Nursing Intervention with a Patient Having a Brain Scan
1. Explain that it is a painless procedure except for the intravenous injection and it only takes a few minutes.
2. Skin testing may be done prior to administration of the isotope.
3. The scanner makes a ticking noise as it moves over the patient.
4. There is no special monitoring of the patient necessary after brain scan.

An *electroencephalogram (EEG)* is a noninvasive test in which electrodes are applied to the scalp to reveal brain wave activity on the surface of the brain. EEG can diagnose seizure disorders, help determine cause of coma, help localize brain lesions, and confirm brain death. During surgery, EEG can monitor brain fuction.

Nursing Intervention with a Patient Having an EEG
1. When possible, wash hair and scalp prior to EEG to allow better electrode contact.
2. Explain that the patient will be asked to relax and remain as quiet as possible during the EEG. Sometimes sedation is necessary. Sometimes the patient may be sleep-deprived the night before.
3. Provide a quiet environment for the test to minimize artifact from surrounding noises and activities.
4. Remove electrode paste from skin and hair after test.
5. If patient routinely takes anticonvulsant drugs, he should check with the physician whether the drug should be stopped prior to the EEG.

The *positron emission tomography (PET scan)* reveals tissues and organ metabolism. Either radioactive gas is inhaled or the patient is injected with a radioactive substance. Positive electrons are emitted from the short-acting radioactive substance and combine with negatively charged electrons from body cells. Emission of gamma rays results, which is seen on a scan. The rate of neuronal metabolic activity and cerebral blood flow can be determined.

Nursing Intervention with a Patient Having a PET Scan
1. Assure patient that there is little exposure to radiation, since the substances used have a short span of activity.
2. The actual test is similar to a CT scan.

A *myelogram* is an invasive diagnostic test in which a contrast material or air is injected into the subarachnoid space either through a lumbar puncture or a cisterna magna puncture.

The patient is strapped to the table and, as it tilts, x-rays are made.

Partial or complete obstruction of the subarachnoid space may be revealed. Bony changes, spinal cord compression, mass, or displacement, abscesses, and ruptured disks may be seen.

The contrast medium used may be water-soluble or oil-based. The water-soluble material does not require displacement of cerebrospinal fluid (CSF), as does the oil-based material. The water-soluble agent is absorbed and does not need to be removed at the end of the procedure as do oil-based agents.

Nursing Intervention with a Patient Having a Myelogram

1. There is some discomfort to the procedure. A local anesthetic will be used for the lumbar puncture.
2. The patient is usually NPO for 4–5 hours before the procedure.
3. Explain the necessity of the tilting of the table during the procedure if an oil-based contrast is used.
4. Pantopaque, an oil-based contrast medium, should not be used in patients with a history of allergic reactions.
5. If an oil-based agent is used, keep the patient's head elevated and observe for meningeal signs postprocedure.
6. If a water-soluble agent is used, keep the patient's head elevated 30–45° for about 6 hours to prevent contact with the cerebral meninges. Watch for nausea, vomiting, and seizures.
7. If air is used, keep the patient's head lower than the trunk so air will move toward the sacral area instead of the head, for 48 hours. If air moves to the head, headache will result.
8. Supply analgesia for headache and antiemetic as necessary postprocedure.

Lumbar puncture (LP) is indicated when a central nervous system (CNS) infection (other than a brain abscess) is suspected, such as meningitis, or it is suspected that there is blood in the subarachnoid space. Some other diseases, such as Guillain-Barré syndrome, may require examination of the cerebrospinal fluid for which a LP is done.

The procedure involves placing a spinal needle at the L2–L3 or L3–L4 levels. Since the spinal cord ends at the L1–L2 vertebral level, it will not be injured. CSF is then allowed to fill a manometer, to measure the opening pressure (normal is 80–180 mm water), and several tubes are filled for examination of the CSF. The CSF is frequently examined for the following:

Color—should be clear. It may be cloudy if white blood cells (WBCs) are elevated, or yellow if old blood pigments are present (xanthrochromic).

Blood—CSF should not be bloody.

Protein—normal value is 15–40 mg/100 ml. Elevated levels may be indicative of Guillain-Barré syndrome, other degenerative diseases, a spinal block, tumor, hemorrhage, or infection.

Glucose—CSF glucose should be ⅔ of the blood glucose. Normal range is 60–80 mg/100 ml. Low levels may indicate an infectious process such as meningitis. High level is not significant.

Cells—CSF should have no more than 5 WBCs per mm. An elevated count may indicate an infectious process or an inflammation within the ventricular system or the meninges.

Electrolytes—sodium, potassium, chloride, calcium, and magnesium are usually checked. Low chloride value may suggest meningitis.

Culture and sensitivity—the organism may be identified and the drug most useful with that specific organism found.

The main danger of LPs is that of herniation of the brain through the tentorial notch or through the foramen magnum. That is the reason for ruling out any space-occupying lesion in the brain prior to doing the LP. If there is increased intracranial pressure, and a needle is placed in the subarachnoid space, suddenly the brain has room to expand, so it expands downward, causing herniation, or a shift of brain into a compartment where it does not belong.

Nursing Intervention with a Patient Having a Lumbar Puncture
1. Explain that a local anesthetic will be used at the needle site. Pressure then may be felt, but not usually pain. Rarely, shooting leg pains may be felt if nerve roots are irritated.
2. Some fear may be relieved by telling the patient that the needle does not enter the spinal cord, so there is no danger of paralysis.
3. Explain the positioning necessary during the exam.
4. Let the patient know the physician may ask him to cough or he may compress the patient's abdomen to be sure the manometer reflects pressure changes with those maneuvers. The patient may also be asked to extend his legs and breathe deeply to ascertain if a high pressure falls with these maneuvers. The physician may also compress the jugular vein on either side of the patient's neck in order to check for obstruction between the spinal needle in the lumbar space and the head.
5. Draw a serum glucose to be able to compare to the CSF glucose value.
6. After the LP, instruct the patient to keep his head flat for 6 to 8 hours to prevent or minimize headache, preferable in prone position to allow the dura to seal.
7. Encourage fluid intake if possible after the procedure to try to replace volume which was removed by the CSF drainage.
8. Watch for CSF leak through puncture site after procedure, or hematoma formation at the site.
9. Check level of consciousness several times after procedure.

Air encephalography is not frequently used since the advent of the CT scan. Pneumoencephalograms and ventriculograms may be useful, however, to identify specific problems in the subarachnoid space or the ventricles, such as obstruction.

A *pneumoencephalogram* involves doing a lumbar puncture while the patient is in a sitting position. Enough CSF is removed and replaced with air or oxygen, so the ventricles fill with the air or oxygen and can be visualized on x-ray with the head in various positions.

Due to the necessity of placing the patient in various positions during this procedure, a pneumoencephalogram is contraindicated in the presence of increased intracranial pressure.

A *ventriculogram* involves a burr hole being made and air or oxygen injected directly into the ventricles, replacing CSF. The procedure is more invasive than the pneumoencephalogram. It can be done on a patient with increased intracranial pressure. The ventricles are well-visualized with this x-ray procedure.

Nursing Intervention with a Patient Having Air Encephalography

Pneumoencephalogram
1. The patient is kept NPO after midnight the evening before the procedure.
2. When air is injected into the subarachnoid space, the patient may have the sensation of air bubbles rising up his back to his head.
3. Postprocedure the head of the bed is kept flat 24 to 48 hours. Vital and neuro signs should be monitored. Fluids should be encouraged to hasten resorption of the air or oxygen.
4. Analgesics for headache and antiemetics may be ordered.
5. Seizure precautions should be maintained.

Ventriculogram
1. The patient's head is shaved in the area of the burr hole.
2. The patient is NPO after midnight the evening before the procedure.
3. Postprocedure care is the same as with pneumoencephalograms.

Electromyography (EMG) records the electrical activity of muscles. Denervation of a muscle and muscle diseases can produce abnormal electrical patterns. Single muscles can also be tested, rather than muscle fibers.

Little needles are placed into the muscle(s) to be tested. Recordings are then made of electrical activity during the time the muscle is at rest and when it is contracting.

Magnetic resonance imaging (MRI) is also called nuclear magnetic resonance. It is a noninvasive test which uses magnetic and radio waves to study the nervous system structures and biochemistry, thus eliminating exposure to radiation. The MRI focuses on the natural atoms in the body. The MRI magnet causes these atoms to align with the external magnetic field.

Nursing Intervention with a Patient Having Electromyography
1. Explain that discomfort will be felt as the needle electrodes are inserted into the muscle(s).
2. Recordings are made with muscles at rest and at work, so the patient will be asked to relax and contract the muscles being tested.

Then the atoms are bombarded with radio waves, deflecting the alignment. Once the radio waves are stopped, a return signal is given which is analyzed by the MRI computer.

MRI is a new diagnostic tool. It may prove helpful in diagnosing stroke, multiple sclerosis, and other cerebrovascular abnormalities.

Nursing Intervention with a Patient Having Magnetic Resonance Imaging
1. Assure patient there is no risk of exposure to radiation.
2. Little to no pre- or postprocedure preparation.

CHAPTER 2

Increased Intracranial Pressure

I. DEFINITION AND DISCUSSION

Intracranial pressure (ICP) is a measure of both static and dynamic forces that influence the volume of intracranial contents. Because the intracranial contents are housed in an essentially closed and rigid skull, when there is an increase of volume, the pressure eventually increases within the skull. The brain has some compensatory mechanisms by which it tries to accommodate the increase in volume inside the skull. Once these mechanisms are exhausted, the pressure rises. Normal ICP is approximately 4–14 mm Hg.

When the intracranial volume expands, perfusion to the brain is compromised. Thus there is an alteration in cerebral tissue perfusion. Deficient perfusion may result in hypoxia, ischemia, and possible infarction of brain tissue.

In the presence of increased intracranial pressure, one might consider the patient to have a decrease in adaptive capacity. The compensatory mechanisms are exhausted and there is very little or no compliance left. The adaptive demand is too great and that patient is not able to adapt to further increases in ICP.

II. ETIOLOGY AND PATHOPHYSIOLOGY

A. Normal Physiology

1. Monro-Kellie Doctrine

—This principle concerning intracranial pressure dynamics states that there are three components inside the enclosed skull. They are brain tissue (approximately 80%), blood (approximately 10%), and cerebrospinal fluid (CSF) (approximately 10%). Volume expansion by any of these three components causes a rise in intracranial pressure if the volume of the other two remains constant.

2. Compensatory Mechanisms

—Compensatory mechanisms allow an increase of some volume within the enclosed skull before the intracranial pressure actually rises.

—Vessels in the head constrict in response to elevated systemic arterial pressure. They dilate in response to a drop in systemic arterial pressure. This is a method of autoregulation, that is, the brain can control the blood supply it receives, in an attempt to keep the perfusion constant.

—Cerebral vessels dilate in response to hypercarbia and hypoxia. This chemical regulation is another mechanism that attempts to assure adequate perfusion for the brain.

—CSF is shunted from the brain to the spinal subarachnoid space in response to an increased volume inside the brain. The lateral ventricles shrink, so much of the CSF volume is shifted from the brain to the spinal subarachnoid space. Normally the volume of CSF within the cranium is about 20 ml, and within the spinal dural sac there is about 140 ml.

—In children before the cranial sutures have fused, there may be expansion of the skull in response to an increased volume inside.

—There may be decreased production of CSF or increased resorption of CSF in response to added intracranial volume.

—The rapidity with which the mass or increase in volume occurs influences the compensation. A small rapidly accumulating mass is less well tolerated than perhaps a larger mass which accumulated slowly. For instance, a slow-growing brain tumor or slow-developing hydrocephalus may be tolerated by a patient for months or years with minimal or no neurologic deficits, because the brain has time to compensate for it. On the other hand, a patient who sustains a sudden head injury, even though the mass is small, such as a small epidural or subdural hemorrhage, may have profound deficits immediately. The brain has had no time to invoke its compensatory mechanisms.

3. Volume-Pressure Relationships

—Once the compensatory mechanisms are exhausted, ICP rises. It is thought that this rise can be plotted on a pressure-volume curve (Fig. 2.1).

—Intracranial compliance refers to the capacity of ICP to adapt to changes in intracranial volume. When compliance is present, the volume-pressure curve rises slowly. A larger volume can be tolerated without a sharp rise in ICP. Once compliance is not operating, the curve rises sharply in response to even a small additional volume to the system.

—A patient may be tested for presence of compliance. It is done by adding a 1 ml bolus of normal saline over one second into an intraventricular catheter or a subarachnoid bolt. If the mean ICP rises greater than 2 mm Hg, the patient is said to have a high volume-pressure response, or minimal compliance. Even small rises in this patient's ICP could be very detrimental, since his response is high on the volume-pressure curve.

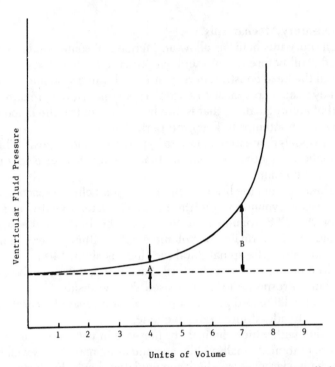

Figure 2.1. Theoretical Pressure-Volume Curve. Note the exponential nature of the curve. Addition of a given volume at point B results in a much greater increase in pressure than the same volume at point A. (Reproduced with permission from Mitchell P: Intracranial hypertension: Implications of research for nursing care," *J Neurosurg Nsg* Sept 1980, p 146.)

4. Cerebral Perfusion Pressure

—Cerebral perfusion pressure (CPP) is equal to the mean arterial blood pressure minus the intracranial pressure. (Mean systemic arterial pressure equals diastolic blood pressure plus one-third pulse pressure.)

—Normal CPP is 80–90 mm Hg.

—Blood flows through the adult brain at a rate of 750 ml/min; 75–80 ml/100 gm/minute of brain tissue in the gray matter and 25 ml/100 gm/minute in the white matter.

—Intracranial blood volume is approximately 200 ml in adults, located mostly in the venous sinuses and in the veins of the pial circulation.

—A decrease in systemic arterial pressure or an increase in ICP lowers CPP.

—A rise in systemic arterial pressure or a drop in ICP raises CPP.

—Cerebral blood flow begins to fail in presence of a CPP of 40 mm Hg.

—Irreversible hypoxic brain damage occurs in presence of a CPP of 30 mm Hg.

—When the ICP and the mean systemic arterial pressure become equal, CPP is zero and there is no blood flow to the brain. The patient may be said to be brain dead.

—Overall cerebral blood flow may be in the normal range, but regional blood flow may be inadequate. A specific region of the brain may become ischemic due to compression of vessels in that area, resulting in clinically evident neurologic deficits, and the ICP may remain normal.

—Autoregulation is the ability of cerebral blood vessels to change their diameter in response to changes in CPP, thus maintaining a constant cerebral blood flow.

—When autoregulation is lost with brain injury, the vessels passively allow volume in the head to follow changes in systemic blood pressure. For example, an increase in systemic blood pressure would cause a rise in ICP, because the vessels are unable to constrict to prevent the rise in cerebral volume and thus ICP.

—Vasomotor paralysis is said to exist when CO_2 reactivity and autoregulation are lost. Cerebral blood flow is truly pressure-passive in this end stage of cerebral decompensation.

5. Venous Outflow

—Most venous outflow from the head is carried by the internal jugular veins. Some is also carried through the basal cerebral venous systems.

—Any activity or position which impedes venous outflow from the head may contribute to an increase volume inside the skull, and thus possibly an increase in ICP.

—Some activities which may decrease venous return are:
• Neck flexion or head rotation to one side.
• Tape from endotracheal tube or tracheostomy ties too tight around the neck.
• Suctioning, coughing, bucking the ventilator, Valsalva maneuver, straining, prone position.
• Use of PEEP (positive end-expiratory pressure) on a ventilator.
• Head of the bed flat.
• Any maneuvers which increase intrathoracic or intraabdominal pressures, such as posturing.
• Hip flexion greater than 90°.

—Cerebral veins have very thin walls with little or no muscle coat. This fact makes the veins susceptible to significant compression before there is any increase in resistance to blood flow, although there is a significant decrease in volume.

B. Pathology

1. Herniation

—Cerebral herniation is a shifting of brain into a compartment where it does not belong. When pressure is elevated in one cranial compartment, brain tissue will protrude into an area of lesser pressure.

—Types of herniation include the following:

a. *Supratentorial Herniation*

Supratentorial types of herniation refer to movement of brain tissue normally situated above the tentorium.

- Cingulate or transfalx herniation occurs when expansion of one hemisphere forces the cingulate gyrus under the falx cerebri laterally. This usually displaces the internal cerebral vein (Fig. 2.2).
- Uncal herniation occurs when a lateral mass forces brain tissue centrally and the uncus (the inner basal medial edge of the temporal lobe) is forced over the tentorial incisura, putting pressure on the brainstem. The earliest sign of uncal herniation may be a moderate unilateral pupil dilatation. The reason for this is that the nuclei of the third cranial nerve, the oculomotor, run bilaterally up the brainstem at the tentorial notch. As pressure is exerted on this third nerve, the outer fibers become compressed. The outer fibers carry parasympathetic innervation to the pupil. The inner fibers are sympathetic fibers. By compressing the parasympathetic fibers, all that is left is sympathetic innervation to the pupil (fight or flight response), thus the pupil dilates.

  As the diencephalon becomes involved, there is a rapid decline in the level of consciousness. Abnormal extensor (decerebrate) response may be demonstrated, initially on the side contralateral to the lesion, and eventually bilaterally. Bilateral Babinski reflexes and Cheyne-Stokes respirations may also appear. Eventually both pupils may become fixed.

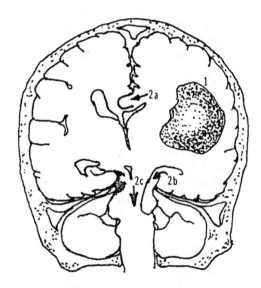

Figure 2.2. Supratentorial herniation. 1 = mass, 2 = herniation. a. cingulate. b. uncal, c. central. (Reproduced with permission from Mauldin R, Coleman L: Intracerebral herniation. *J Neurosurg Nsg* Oct 1983, p 288.)

- Central or transentorial herniation occurs when there is diffuse, gen-eralized pressure in the area above the tentorium. Such a diffuse pres-sure is commonly exerted by blood in the subarachnoid space. Pressure occurs in a rostral-caudal direction. As pressure is put upon the dien-cephalon, the thalamus, hypothalamus, subthalamus, and/or epithalamus may all get pushed through the tentorial opening. An early sign of this occurrence is a decrease in level of consciousness. Initially the pupils are small and briskly reactive to light. The patient may yawn and sigh deeply or have Cheyne-Stokes breathing. As the herniation progresses the pupils become fixed and dilated, Babinski reflexes are present bilater-ally, flaccidity occurs, and respiration and blood pressure fall. Bilateral motor involvement is expected, because the pressure is diffuse and thus usually equal on both sides.

b. *Infratentorial or Subtentorial Herniation*
Infratentorial types of herniation refer to those in which brain tissue beneath the tentorium is moved into an abnormal compartment. Because this area of the brain is closer to the lower brainstem, controlling vital functions, the progression may be more rapid and more likely to be fatal.

Infratentorial herniation may involve protrusion of tissue, usually a tonsil (tip of the cerebellum closest to the foramen magnum) downward through the foramen magnum (Fig. 2.3). This is called a tonsilar or foramen

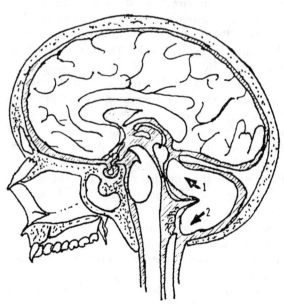

Figure 2.3. Infratentorial herniation. 1 = upward, 2 = downward. (Reproduced with permission from Mauldin R, Coleman L: Intracerebral herniation. *J Neurosurg Nsg* Oct 1983, p 288.)

magnum herniation. There may also be upward herniation in which infratentorial tissue is pushed upward through the tentorium.

Infratentorial herniation may be a result of a cerebellar tumor, abscess, hemorrhage, brainstem lesions, or insertion of a needle into the subarachnoid space during a lumbar puncture when there is increased ICP in the supratentorial area.

Clinically, asymmetrical signs of focal brainstem disorder are usually seen with infratentorial herniation. There is usually rapid loss of consciousness. Other signs may depend on the level of brainstem involvement. For example, with injury at the midbrain level, pupils may be fixed at midposition. Lower pontine injury may be reflected with miotic pupils which are reactive to light.

c. *Transcalvarian Herniation*
Transcalvarian herniation refers to protrusion of brain tissue to the outside of the skull. The usual cause is a penetrating head injury, such as a gunshot wound to the head. It may also occur through a craniotomy site over which the bone flap has not been replaced.

2. Signs and Symptoms of Increased Intracranial Pressure

—Change in level of consciousness is usually the earliest clinical sign seen as intracranial pressure rises. The reticular activating system (RAS) receives input from all sense organs and from higher centers in the brain. This input is sent to the cortex in a continuous bombardment, stimulating the cortex. The RAS is considered our center for consciousness. It determines whether we are alert or unconscious. As ICP increases, stimulation of the cortex is diminished, thus causing the patient to be less awake. This is the change in level of consciousness we see clinically.

—Change in motor and sensory function may be seen as a result of pressure on a specific area of the brain (see Chapter 1). Extension (decerebrate) or flexion (decorticate) posturing may be seen.

—Any pupil change that is a change from a specific patient's baseline may be significant. A blown pupil is a unilateral fixed and dilated pupil, possibly indicating ipsilateral uncal herniation. However, a pupil does not have to become blown to indicate deterioration in the neurologic status of a patient. Small reactive pupils may indicate the same level of deterioration if it is a change from baseline.

—Changes in vital signs may occur, but are late signs (see Chapter 1). There may be a widened pulse pressure and bradycardia.

—Abnormal reflexes such as a Babinski may be present. Brainstem reflexes may be lost with increased ICP.

—Headache is not an usual symptom of increased ICP, since the cortex has no pain receptors. However, when the meningeal arteries, venous sinuses, or arteries and dura mater at the base of the brain are compressed, headache

may result, since they do have pain receptors. Morning headaches are often associated with brain tumors.
—Vomiting may be seen as the increased ICP causes ischemia in the medulla (the emetic center).
—Papilledema is a swelling of the optic disk, resulting from pressure on the optic nerve, thus impeding venous return from the retina. It may not be an early sign of increasing ICP.
—Elevation of the bone flap site may be seen if the patient has had a craniotomy and a piece of the skull has been left off to allow for swelling. There may be visible bulging at the craniectomy defect.
—Dysrhythmias may occur as ICP rises.
—If a lumbar puncture is done, there may be an elevated opening pressure. A lumbar puncture is contraindicated if a mass effect is suspected in the head, for fear of causing a herniation.
—Seizures may result.

3. Types of Brain Edema

Brain edema is often, but not always, associated with increased intracranial pressure. It reduces intracranial compliance before it raises the ICP. Brain edema does contribute to morbidity and mortality of many patients.

a. *Vasogenic (extracellular) edema*
   —Located primarily in the white matter.
   —Most common form of brain edema.
   —Involves increased capillary permeability to large molecules, thus allowing the serum content (such as the plasma proteins) to leak across the capillary wall into the brain tissue. This causes an increase in extracellular fluid volume.
   —There are an increased number of pinocytes, which are cells in the systemic capillaries that help with transport of large molecules across the capillaries. This is significant because large molecules can travel from the capillaries through the blood-brain barrier by active transport. The normally tight junctions of the blood-brain barrier are impaired so that fluid from within the capillary flows out into the brain tissue.
   —Some conditions that may result in vasogenic brain edema are brain tumors, head trauma or hemorrhage, cerebral infarction, abscesses and postcraniotomy.
   —Influenced greatly by systolic blood pressure. If systolic pressure is high in the capillaries, more vascular fluid will be pushed out into the brain tissue through the damaged blood-brain barrier.

b. *Cytotoxic (intracellular) brain edema*
   —Occurs in both white and gray matter.
   —Blood-brain barrier remains intact.
   —Involves swelling of the brain cells, including the neurons, glia, and endothelial cells within the capillaries.

—As swelling occurs inside the cell, the extracellular fluid space diminishes. There is an increase in intracellular water and sodium.

—This type of edema is triggered by a disturbance of the cellular metabolism. This affects the sodium pump of the cells, and the active ion transport. The impaired aerobic cellular metabolism results in the brain quickly using the available oxygen and glucose and then converting to anaerobic metabolism. Anaerobic metabolism does not produce enough energy to maintain the energy-dependent sodium pump within the cells. So sodium and water begin to accumulate within the cell, causing it eventually to break down inside them. When breakdown occurs, the osmolarity inside the cell increases, pulling in yet more fluid, and thus more swelling occurs.

—Some conditions that may result in cytotoxic brain edema are hypoxia or anoxia such as from cardiac arrest, water intoxication, Reye's syndrome, ischemia, and hypoosmolality.

c. *Interstitial (hydrocephalic) brain edema*

—Occurs primarily in the periventricular white matter.

—Occurs when there is an increase in CSF pressure within the ventricles. The CSF is pushed out of the ventricles across the ependymal cells that line the ventricles, into the periventricular spaces. So the edema fluid is mostly CSF.

—The extracellular fluid space and volume increases as the CSF is forced out of the ventricles.

—Symptoms of this type of edema may be reversed with a shunting procedure if done early. If not treated, gait disturbances and dementia result.

—Some conditions that may result in interstitial brain edema are obstructive hydrocephalus and pseudotumor cerebri.

III. GENERAL TREATMENT

A. Medical Management of Increased ICP

1. Hyperventilation

Hyperventilation should keep the $PaCO_2$ at 25–28 mm Hg, stimulating cerebral vasoconstriction. In order to accomplish hyperventilation, a pH of up to 7.55 is acceptable. If the pH rises much above this level, the oxygen-hemoglobin dissociation curve shifts to the left. This results in the hemoglobin not releasing the oxygen to the brain tissue. Seizures may also result from alkalemia. The PaO_2 should be kept over 80 mm Hg.

—There is much controversy over the length of time during which hyperventilation is beneficial. Some researchers claim that renal mechanisms compensate for respiratory alkalosis after 48 to 72 hours, returning cerebral blood flow to normal. One method of determining whether the patient is still being benefited by hyperventilation is to allow the $PaCO_2$ to resume normal levels. If the ICP rises during this normalizing procedure, reinstitute the hyperventilation. If the ICP drops in response to the hyperventilation, then it is obviously benefiting the patient.

2. Osmotic Diuretics

—Mannitol is usually chosen over the use of urea for the following reasons:
- Onset of action for Mannitol is faster (15–30 minutes versus 1–2 hours for urea).
- Urea is inconvenient to mix, since it is not in liquified form, ready to administer.
- Urea is unstable in solution, and should be discarded after 8 hours.

—Osmotic diuretics pull water out of healthy brain tissue and deposit it in the cardiovascular system. So the cardiovascular system should be assessed prior to administration to prevent pulmonary edema.

—Mannitol establishes an osmotic gradient across the blood-brain barrier which depletes the intracellular and extracellular fluid volume within the brain and throughout the body.

—Mannitol is also thought to decrease production of CSF, which helps to reduce the ICP.

—Diuresis of water may cause a systemic dehydration, so electrolytes and serum osmolarity must be monitored. Cardiac dysrhythmias may also result.

—Other side effects of Mannitol administration may include hypotension, tachycardia, hemoconcentration.

—Usual dose of Mannitol is 1–3 gm/kg of body weight given intravenously.

—There is a rebound effect of Mannitol. Normally, Mannitol does not cross the blood-brain barrier. So it provides its therapeutic effect in healthy brain tissue, where the blood-brain barrier is intact and there are normal capillaries and cell membranes. However, with some head injuries, the blood-brain barrier becomes leaky, so there is increased capillary permeability. In these areas Mannitol may permeate the blood-brain barrier and reverse the therapeutic osmotic gradient, making the brain side more concentrated than the blood side of the barrier. This gradient then will produce a condition where water is pulled into the brain, increasing the swelling.

Some neurosurgeons feel that the amount of swelling caused by the rebound is greater than that prior to administration of the Mannitol. So those physicians may elect to use Mannitol only in a situation where they need some time to get to the operating room to repair an operable lesion.

—Mannitol should be given with a .45 micron filter.

—Mannitol is usually contraindicated if there is an active intracranial bleed. By reducing cerebral volume, the bleeding could be increased or a new hemorrhage precipitated.

—If the entire brain is grossly damaged, and there are few or no normal capillaries and cell membranes, hypertonic solutions such as Mannitol are ineffective. This is true in presence of vasogenic edema.

3. Corticosteroids

—Dexamethasone (Decadron) is often the steroid of choice because of its lower sodium-retaining properties.

—There is much controversy over the effectiveness of steroids in treating increased intracranial pressure and most head injuries. If used, they should be administered early in the course of treatment, since they are not fast-acting, and the therapeutic effects will not be seen immediately. Onset of action for dexamethasone is 12 to 24 hours.

—If steroids have been administered for a week or more, they should be tapered and not discontinued abruptly. The adrenal glands need some time to begin functioning efficiently again after being depressed by the steroid treatment. Adrenocortical insufficiency may result if steroids are discontinued quickly.

—Steroids are thought to make the gastric mucosa more permeable to hydrochloric acid, so to prevent gastrointestinal distress and possible bleeding, antacids or cimetadine (Tagamet) are usually given as long as the patient is receiving steroids.

—Steroids may mask an infectious process, elevate blood pressure, and elevate serum glucose levels.

—Mechanism of action is not fully understood, but it is believed that dexamethasone may stabilize cell membranes and repair a leaky blood-brain barrier, as well as increase resorption of CSF.

—Usefulness of dexamethasone in controlling brain swelling may be impaired by phenytoin (Dilantin), since it increases the metabolism and excretion of dexamethasone.

4. Hypothermia

—ICP increases with hyperpyrexia.

—Each one degree Centigrade rise in temperature increases the metabolic demands of the brain by approximately 10%.

—Hypothermia reduces brain metabolism, making it less vulnerable to hypoxia.

—Hypothermia may be achieved with cooling blankets and antipyretics.

—Shivering must be prevented, so chlorpromazine may be given.

5. Fluid Management

—Fluid restriction is usually imposed in the range of 1000–1500 ml/24 hrs. There is some debate about the degree of dehydration which should be achieved. Some authorities believe a severe fluid restriction causes hypovolemia, which reduces cerebral perfusion, and this is detrimental to the patient.

—Dextrose in water is usually avoided, and some intravenous solution with saline in it is used to prevent hemodilution and exacerbation of cerebral edema.

—A nasogastric tube is necessary during coma, since the gastrointestinal tract is depressed. The volume of gastric aspirate may be replaced with i.v. fluid.

—Accurate intake and output is necessary.

6. Furosemide (Lasix)

—Furosemide may be used in conjunction with an osmotic diuretic to facilitate the patient's getting rid of the water which was pulled from the brain and deposited in the cardiovascular system. This may help prevent pulmonary edema, especially in a patient with some compromise of his cardiovascular status.

—Serum electrolytes are monitored and replaced as necessary. The serum sodium is especially important to keep in the high-normal range. If hyponatremia develops, the injured brain side of the blood-brain barrier becomes more concentrated than the serum, and water will be pulled into the brain to equalize the osmotic gradients.

7. Barbiturate Coma

—Barbiturate coma is usually used for a severe refractory ICP over 40 mm Hg or for a persistent increased ICP despite aggressive therapy and in the presence of a deteriorating neurologic status.

—Barbiturates may be used to lower ICP by reducing the metabolic demands of the brain, allowing for healing to occur. It is thought by some that barbiturates may improve neuronal survival in the ischemic brain tissue, making the injured brain less susceptible to hypoxia.

—Barbiturates reduce systemic blood pressure, which reduces hydrostatic pressure in the injured brain tissue and helps relieve edema.

—Hypotension caused by the barbiturate may be treated with dopamine if necessary.

—Barbiturates reduce cerebral metabolism by reducing the functional electrical generation of the neurons. This is the reason an isoelectric (flat) EEG may be seen in patients in a barbiturate coma.

Potential Complications of Barbiturate Coma:
1. Protective reflexes are lost, such as gag, swallow, and corneals.
2. The immobile patient is prone to development of stasis of pulmonary secretions, increased cardiac workload, thrombus formation, skin breakdown, urinary status, and contractures.
3. Multiple invasive monitoring lines put the patient at risk for infection.
4. Peristalsis is slowed or stopped during therapy, so nutritional needs may have to be met with hyperalimentation.
5. Body temperature may not adequately reflect presence or absence of sepsis during barbiturate coma.

—Barbiturates cause muscle relaxation and thus cerebral venous pressure is reduced.

—Barbiturates act as an anticonvulsant.

—When the ICP has remained normal (usually below 20 mm Hg) for 24 to 72 hours, the barbiturates may be gradually tapered over one to several days. If, however, the ICP again increases, treatment is often reinstituted. Adults may be especially difficult to bring out of coma without their ICP elevating. Children seem to respond better to this therapy, especially those with Reye's syndrome.

—As the barbiturate coma is relieved, it is recommended that the patient have a therapeutic serum level of phenytoin, to prevent withdrawal seizures.

Recommendations for Instituting Barbiturate Coma:

1. A knowledgeable intensive care team.
2. An intracranial pressure monitoring device is necessary, since the coma will obliterate clinical assessment parameters ordinarily used to assess neurologic status. Even brainstem responses, including oculocephalic and oculovestibular, are absent. Brainstem auditory evoked responses do remain intact.
3. Arterial pressure monitoring is recommended. CPP may be calculated from the mean arterial pressure readings.
4. A pulmonary artery line is recommended since barbiturates can change blood pressure and depress the myocardium. So a hemodynamic assessment tool is recommended. Cardiac output, central venous pressure, and fluid volume status can thus be monitored.
5. Cardiac monitoring.
6. Controlled ventilation.
7. A laboratory able to give rapid results of barbiturate levels.
8. An available CT scanner is recommended.

—Muscle weakness resulting from lack of use during barbiturate coma often prolongs the length of time required to return a patient to adequate unassisted ventilation.

—Since barbiturates are metabolized by the liver and excreted by the kidneys, impaired liver and/or kidney function may significantly alter the ability to attain, maintain, and reduce the serum barbiturate level. Liver function tests should be monitored during barbiturate coma.

8. Phenytoin (Dilantin)

—May be given to prevent seizures, which could cause an increase in the brain's metabolism and make it more susceptible to hypoxia.

—Contraindicated in patients with heart block, sinus bradycardia, and Stokes-Adams syndrome.

9. Ventriculostomy Drainage
—CSF may be drained from the subarachnoid space to reduce ICP. Parameters may be established so that either nurses can intermittently drain off CSF if the ICP is greater than a predetermined measurement, or a system of automatic siphoning of CSF may be established.

10. Surgical Management
—If there is a surgically accessible lesion, its removal may reduce ICP.

11. Lidocaine
—Lidocaine as a drug for treating intracranial hypertension is still rather experimental, with inconsistent results.

12. Patient Positioning
—Head of the bed elevated.
—Head in neutral alignment without neck flexion or head rotation.
—Hip flexion over 90° is avoided.

13. Discussion around the Patient's Bed
—Avoid discussion over the patient's bed about him or his prognosis.
—Avoid saying aloud anything around the patient which you would not say to him were he awake.

14. Paralyzing Agents
—Pavulon or another paralyzing agent may be needed to control ICP if the patient has severe decerebrate (extensor) or decorticate (flexor) posturing. These positions increase intrathoracic pressure, which compromises venous return from the head.

15. Miscellaneous Measures
—Painful stimulation may increase cerebral blood flow, which raises ICP. So this may be a detrimental tool to use to assess neurologic status.
—If positive end-expiratory pressure (PEEP) over 8 cm of water is necessary on the ventilator, it will impede cerebral venous outflow. The value of the PEEP for a pulmonary problem may need to be weighed against the detrimental effect of the elevated ICP.

B. Diagnostic Tests
—The CT scan will provide information about a possible operative lesion, if that is the cause of the increased ICP. It will indicate brain swelling and a shift of the lateral ventricles, if present.
—Sensory evoked potentials, such as brainstem auditory evoked responses, may be used to evaluate the integrity of the brainstem.
—Doppler ultrasonographic evaluation of cerebral blood flow may be done to evaluate total hemispheric blood flows.
—An angiogram may provide information about the patency of the cerebral circulation.

—A regional cerebral blood flow study may be done to estimate brain perfusion. There is evidence indicating that blood flow through brain tissue is directly related to the tissue's metabolic needs. So if brain perfusion is indicative of the metabolism of the brain, that too may be studied with this noninvasive test. The patient breathes radioactive xenon gas and the radioactive clearance from the brain is measured.

—A brain flow study may be used to determine brain death. When no cerebral blood flow is seen, the brain is receiving no perfusion.

—Magnetic resonance imaging may indicate brain swelling and possible herniation, if present.

—Intracranial pressure monitoring may be considered a diagnostic tool, and sometimes a therapuetic measure as well. There are several methods of monitoring ICP:

- Ventricular catheter monitoring
    1. A burr hole is made, usually in the patient's nondominant hemisphere and a small catheter is threaded into one of the lateral ventricles.
    2. If swelling has already occurred, it may be difficult for the physician to find the collapsed or decompressed ventricle.
    3. The catheter allows drainage of CSF from the ventricular system that may quickly alleviate a high ICP. It also allows sampling of CSF for laboratory examination.
    4. Risk of infection is significant since it is very invasive, penetrating the cerebrum. Percutaneous tunneling of the catheter may reduce the possibility for infection.
    5. Volume-pressure response may be measured, (see page 21).
- Subarachnoid screw monitoring
    1. A screw is placed via burr hole into the subarachnoid space on the patient's nondominant side.
    2. For accurate readings, the skull should be intact.
    3. Ease of insertion may be more than with a ventricular catheter if the ventricular system is collapsed.
    4. Not as easy to withdraw CSF from a bolt (screw) as from the ventricular catheter.
    5. Volume-pressure response measurements possible.
- Epidural sensor monitoring
    1. A fiber-optic sensor is inserted into the epidural space via a burr hole.
    2. Least invasive method of monitoring since the dura is not penetrated.
    3. Least accurate method, because it is not measuring ICP directly from a cranial space filled with CSF. Readings may run 1–2 mm Hg higher than ventricular catheter readings.
    4. Unable to withdraw CSF.
    5. Sensor will not become obstructed with brain tissue or blood, as can happen with the catheter and the screw.

6. Unable to check the readings of the system with a water manometer.
7. Volume-pressure response testing not possible.
- Subdural monitoring
  1. A three-way stopcock is placed into the subdural space with a twist drill.
  2. No direct access to the CSF, so volume-pressure response measurements are not feasible, and no opportunity to sample or withdraw CSF.
  3. Easy to insert.
—ICP waveform interpretation (Fig. 2.4).
- A normal ICP waveform has a steep upward slope followed by a downward slope with a dicrotic notch. Normal ICP ranges between 4–15 mm Hg. Some of the newer research indicates we should treat an ICP of 15 mm Hg rather than 20 mm, which has most often been our cutoff up until now.
- A waves (plateau waves, Lundberg waves) are the most harmful and clinically significant.
  1. Considered an indication of intracranial decompensation.
  2. Elevate to levels of 50–100 mm Hg.
  3. Duration of elevation may be 5–20 minutes.
  4. Tend to occur in patients with existing elevations in ICP (20–40 mm Hg).
  5. Often accompanied by temporary increase in neurologic deficits.
  6. Significant because they reduce CPP and contribute to brain cell hypoxia and possibly irreversible brain damage.
- B waves
  1. Not thought to be clinically significant because the elevation in pressure is not sustained. They may occur more frequently with reduced intracranial compliance.
  2. Frequency of spike is every 1½–2 minutes.
  3. May reach pressures of 50 mm Hg.
  4. Often related to changes in respiration, as in Cheyne-Stokes breathing. Mechanism may be influenced by changes in intrathoracic pressure or fluctuations of $PaCO_2$ due to the breathing pattern.
- C waves
  1. Not clinically significant because the elevated pressure is not sustained.
  2. Frequency of spike is every 1–2 minutes.
  3. May reach pressures of 20–50 mm Hg.
  4. May be related to respirations or changes in blood pressure.
- Some treatment protocols call for treatment of a single wave spike if it is over 30 mm Hg. Others treat a continuous rise in ICP.

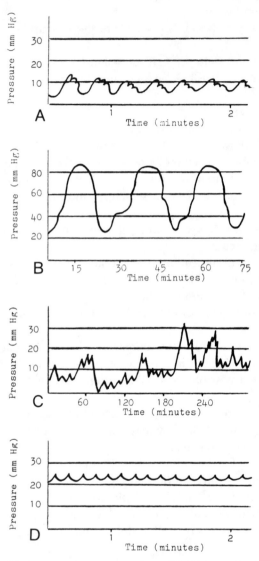

Figure 2.4. *A,* Normal ICP Waveform. *B,* A waves. *C,* B waves. *D,* C waves. (Reproduced with permission from Smith S: Continuous intracranial pressure monitoring: implications and applications for critical care. *Critical Care Nurse* 3(4):45 1983.)

C. Special Nursing Measures

—Draining cerebrospinal fluid from a ventriculostomy should be done slowly. Rapid decompression of the ventricles may cause the bridging cortical veins to tear, creating a subdural hemorrhage.

—There are currently no infection control recommendations from the Cen-

---

Nursing Management
Nursing priorities for care of a patient with increased ICP.
1. Ensure adequate respiratory function:
2. Recognize and respond to early signs of increased ICP.
3. Manage pain.
4. Provide patient/family with information regarding support groups/resources available.

Nursing Diagnoses most frequently associated with increased ICP:
—Ineffective breathing patterns related to altered level of consciousness, immobility.
—Alteration in tissue perfusion: cerebral related to hypervolemia/hypovolemia, changes in blood pressure, interruption of arterial/venous blood flow, decreased cardiac output, dysrhythmias, intracerebral steal, loss of intracranial compliance, hemorrhage.
—Alteration in fluid volume: excess related to neuro/hormonal dysfunction, side effects of drugs.
—Fluid volume deficit related to side effects of drugs such as osmotic diuretics, fluid restriction neuro/hormonal dysfunction.
—Alteration in pattern of urinary elimination related to immobility, inability to verbalize needs, indwelling catheter.
—Impairment of skin integrity related to immobility, invasive catheters.
—Potential for infection related to immunosuppression, compromised nutrition status, depressed respiratory function, drug therapy, immobility, impaired skin integrity (e.g., insertion of tubes and catheters, invasive procedures).
—Impaired physical mobility related to altered level of consciousness, enforced bedrest, neurologic deficit, weakness.
—Alteration in nutrition: less than body requirements related to altered level of consciousness, oral intake restriction, increased energy expenditure, decreased peristalsis.
—Alteration in bowel elimination: incontinence related to depressed level of consciousness, cognitive deficit, muscle weakness, inability to verbalize needs, enforced bedrest.
—Self-care deficit: total related to altered level of consciousness.
—Impaired communication: verbal related to intubation, tracheostomy, neurologic deficit, brain damage.
—Alteration in oral mucous membrane related to fluid restriction, dehydration, immunosuppression, invasive procedures, inadequate oral hygiene, malnutrition.
—Knowledge deficit regarding the condition, treatment, expected outcomes.

ters for Disease Control (CDC) with regard to ICP care. The fewer stop-cocks in the monitoring system, the less risk for introducing organisms into the system. Some physicians prefer an antibiotic in the flush solution, but studies have not demonstrated less infection with the antibiotic than with a normal saline flush solution. There are no recommendations about the frequency of dressing changes or tubing changes in the ICP set up. The flush solution should be changed every 24 hours, according to CDC recommendations for i.v. solution changes.

—Do not use normal saline in the multidose vial for irrigating an ICP device. It contains an alcohol preservative which is irritating to the meninges. Use the i.v. solution normal saline.

—Routine withdrawal of CSF for culture may be ordered for early detection of infection.

—The zero point of the ICP monitor should be releveled after every position change of the patient or at least every eight hours. The range of numbers for monitoring ICP is low, so a reading which is even 2–3 mm Hg in error may be significant, and cause the patient to be treated or not treated.

—A volume-measure i.v. set (volutrole, metriset, buretrol) using a minidripper is recommended for use on patients with acute head injuries or labile ICP's. These patients may herniate with the rapid addition of even a small amount of fluid. Thus, running i.v. fluid from a volume-measure set gives the caregiver more control over fluid infusion. If the intravenous catheter is in a positional site a patient could conceivably receive a liter of fluid very rapidly without a volume-measure set in line.

—When giving Mannitol, check for crystalization in the bottle before administering. If crystals are present, they may be dissolved by placing the bottle in warm water.

—Patients receiving osmotic diuretics should be weighed daily.

—If administering phenytoin (Dilantin) intravenously, the patient should be on a cardiac monitor. Too rapid administration may cause cardiac arrest. Watch the monitor during administration for prolonged P-R intervals and signs of heart block. It is recommended that 40 mg/minute should be the maximal infusion rate. If a patient will be receiving phenytoin on a long-term basis, good oral hygiene should be taught to minimize gum disorders.

SUGGESTED READINGS

Burgess K: Recognizing and responding to increased ICP. *Nursing Life* 5(2):34–48, 1985.
Mauldin R, Coleman L: Intracerebral herniation. *J Neurosurg Nursing* 15(5):287–290, 1983.
McNamara M, Quinn C: Epidural intracranial pressure monitoring: Theory and clinical application. *J Neurosurg Nursing* 13(5): 267–281, 1981.
Mitchell P: Intracranial hypertension: Implications of research for nursing care. *J Neurosurg Nursing* 12(3): 145–154, 1980.
Smith S: Continuous intracranial pressure monitoring: Implications and applications for critical care. *Crit Care Nurse* 3(4): 42–51, 1983.
Speers, I: Cerebral edema. *J Neurosurg Nursing* 13(2): 102–115, 1981.

CHAPTER 3

Head Trauma

I. DEFINITION AND DISCUSSION

Victims of head trauma may demonstrate more than alterations in thought processes. If the injury resulted in a motor deficit, such as a hemiparesis or hemiplegia, there will be impaired physical mobility and perhaps a selfcare deficit (see Chapter 5). The motor deficit may put the patient at risk for injury. Feedback and warnings about the potential for injury may not be utilized or incorporated due to the altered thought processes and lack of understanding.

Depending on where the brain is injured, there may be impaired verbal communication (see Chapter 5). Other methods of communication may need to be developed. Retraining may lessen the impaired verbal communication. The communication, once established, may contain inappropriate content, since the thought processes are altered.

So it is not one area of the head-injured patient's life that is changed. The alteration in thought processes may contribute to potential problems in other areas of daily living.

A. General Information

—Trauma is currently the third most common cause of death in the United States, and frequently the patient sustains a head injury (neurotrauma).
—Every 16 seconds a head injury occurs to someone across the United States.
—Approximately 60,000 to 75,000 individuals suffer moderate head injuries which render them disabled for more than 3 months.
—Over 500,000 Americans sustain minor head injuries each year. More than 290,000 people are hospitalized for minor head trauma. Of the minor head injuries, some 150,000 will suffer some disability for one month or more.
—Each year more than 140,000 Americans die as a result of head injuries. Head injury kills more Americans under the age of 34 than *all other causes* combined. (From National Head Injury Foundation, Inc., Southborough, MA.)

—The leading cause of head trauma is motor vehicle accidents. Contributing factors are alcohol consumption and seat belt noncompliance.
—A study from a regional CNS (central nervous system) trauma center in Virginia made these findings:
  • Forty per cent of head injured patients had previously been hospitalized for a head injury;
  • Males were victims of head trauma in a 3:1 ratio to females;
  • Eighty-five per cent of their head-injured patients had been drinking;
  • Most often, it was the driver who was injured, not the passenger;
  • Most were involved in single car accidents.
—Mortality with head trauma is highest when due to violence (e.g., gunshot wounds), and second highest with auto accidents.
—Head injuries are the primary cause of death in patients under 45 years of age.
—Head trauma may result in long-term deficits in thought processing as well as impaired physical mobility.

B. Pathophysiology
—Most of the pathophysiology of head trauma is based on the principles of increasing intracranial pressure (see Chapter 2).

C. Classification of Head Injuries

Concussion
—No structural break in the skull or dura.
—No residual neurodeficits.
—If the patient becomes unconscious it is for 5 minutes or less.
—Brain shows no visible damage.
—A rise in ICP (intracranial pressure) may occur with subsequent pressure put on the brainstem.
—One theory is that excessive acetylcholine is released following brain injury, and that this in some way interferes with transmission of nerve impulses.

Contusion (Fig. 3.1)
—Closed head injury to the brain with small diffuse venous hemorrhage.
—Both white and gray matter may be bruised and discolored.
—There may be prolonged unconsciousness and immediate neurodeficits, with deterioration in level of consciousness.
—Contusions are most frequently found near bony prominences of the skull. The brainstem may be injured.
—May result in permanent tissue damage and scarring. Residual deficits depend on location and severity of injury.

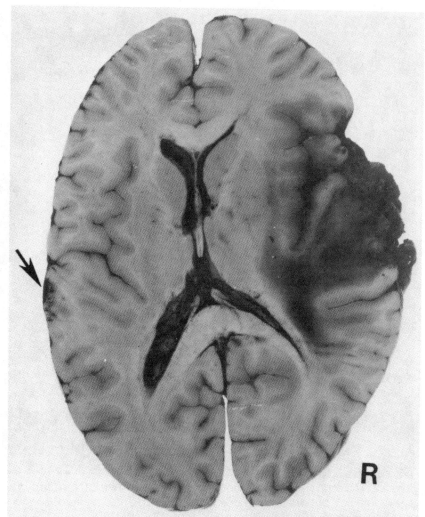

Figure 3.1.   Cross-section of a recently traumatized brain showing a large temporal contusion on the right and a smaller contusion on the left (*arrow*). (Reproduced with permission from Cooper PR (ed): *Head Injury*. Baltimore, Williams & Wilkins, 1982, p 239.)

Epidural Hemorrhage (Extradurals) (Fig. 3.2)
—Thirty per cent mortality rate.
—Usually due to arterial bleed associated with a skull fracture.
—Usually due to nick in the middle meningeal artery, in groove of temporal bone.
—Anatomically, where the skull is covered with many muscles, such as the

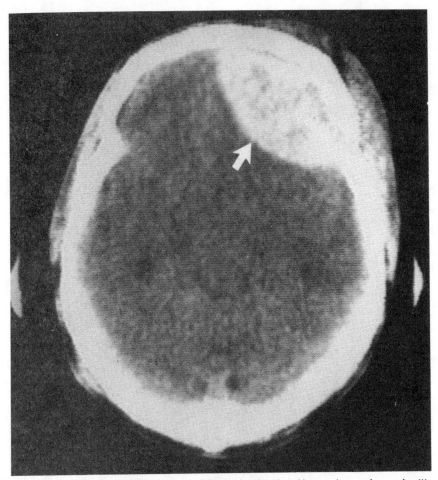

Figure 3.2. CT scan showing large left frontal extradural hematoma (*arrow*) with typical lentiform appearance. (Reproduced with permission from Cooper PR (ed): *Head Injury.* Baltimore, Williams & Wilkins, 1982, p 239.)

back of the neck and in front of the ears (chewing muscles), the skull beneath is thin. Where there is little muscle coverage, the skull is thicker for protection. The chewing muscles cover the area where the middle meningeal artery runs, so the bone beneath is quite thin. Thus a blow to this area often damages this artery, causing an epidural hemorrhage.

—Patient may deteriorate faster than one with a subdural hemorrhage because it involves an arterial rather than a venous bleed.

—Classically, the patient has a transient loss of consciousness, wakes up, and then loses consciousness again.

—Treatment involves surgical evacuation. It cannot be absorbed nor encapsulated.

—Bleeding is initially stopped by tamponade effect of the clot against the brain and the bleeding vessel. Thus it is dangerous to give the patient Mannitol or any agent which would decrease swelling, thus relieving the tamponade effect, allowing the vessel to rebleed.

—Occurs in about 2% of head-injured patients.

—Effects children and adolescents more often than adults because dura isn't yet attached firmly to the bony table.

Subdural Hemorrhage (Fig. 3.3)

—Usually is a venous bleed. Cortical veins in the space between the dura and the arachnoid are damaged, and blood slowly seeps from them. Normally, there is only a small amount of a lymph-like material in the subdural space.

—Occurs in 10% to 15% of head injuries.

—The elderly and the chronic alcoholic populations may have cerebral atrophy, creating a larger subdural space, with lack of support for the venous network. Therefore, trauma to the head is more likely to result in a subdural hemorrhage. Another population at higher than normal risk for developing a subdural is patients on anticoagulants. Following minor trauma, a damaged vessel will normally seal the defect by clot formation. Anticoagulant therapy delays this process.

1. **Acute subdurals**
   - Symptoms occur quickly, within 24 hours.
   - Focal signs may include hemiparesis or hemiplegia, confusion, headache, lethargy or agitation.
   - The brain is unable to tolerate rapid compression. Surgical removal of the clot is necessary by formal craniotomy.
   - Postoperatively, the head of the bed should be elevated to enhance venous outflow from the head.

2. **Chronic subdurals**
   - Blood in the subdural space eventually becomes encapsulated by the dura as the red blood cells hemolyze and blood proteins disintegrate in a week or so, the osmotic concentration within the encapsulated clot becomes elevated, drawing in water from the surrounding area. Thus the clot becomes liquified over time, which makes it easier to evacuate. Burr holes may be used instead of a craniotomy, thus reducing morbidity and mortality from more complicated surgery (Fig. 3.4).
   - Symptoms may not show up for weeks, depending on the amount of cerebral atrophy present.
   - Postoperatively, the head of the bed should be kept flat to allow gravity to help the healthy brain expand to fill the evacuation site. Sometimes a subdural drain may be placed during surgery. The patient's head should

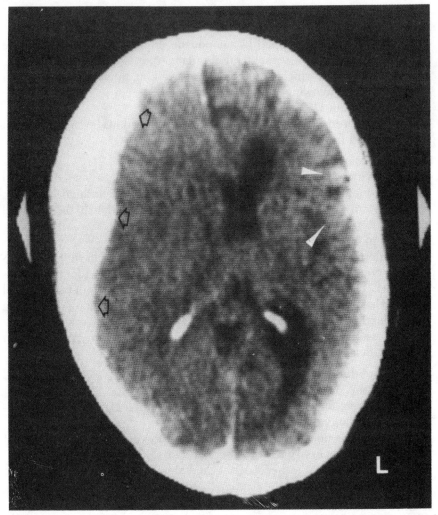

Figure 3.3. CT scan showing acute right subdural hematoma (*black arrows*) with compression and right to left shift of right lateral ventricle. *Arrowheads* identify left-sided cerebral contusion. (Reproduced with permission from Cooper PR (ed): *Head Injury*. Baltimore, Williams & Wilkins, 1982, p 190.)

remain flat while the drain is in place, and for 24 hours after it is removed to prevent air being pulled into the subdural space.

- Physicians may allow an acute subdural hematoma to become chronic for easier evacuation if the patient is not demonstrating severe neurologic deficits.
- Symptoms of a chronic subdural may include headache, lethargy, confusion, slowness of thought processes, and coma.

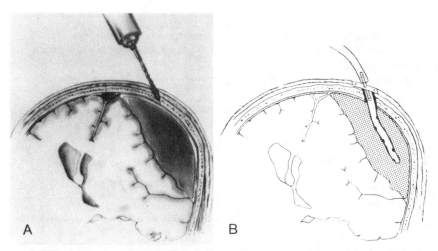

Figure 3.4. A, Drawing demonstrates how a twist drill hole is made at an oblique angle to the skull over the site of maximum thickness of a chronic subdural hematoma. B, a rubber catheter is passed into the subdural space through the twist drill hole for evacuation of liquefied chronic subdural hematoma. (Reproduced with permission from Tabaddor K, Shulman K: Definitive treatment of chronic subdural hematoma by twist-drill craniostomy and closed-system drainage. J Neurosurg 46:220–226, 1977.)

Subarachnoid Hemorrhage (SAH)
—About ⅔ of the victims survive the initial bleeding. The other ⅓ die within the first 24–48 hours after hemorrhage.
—There is usually little or no warning of onset.
—Classically its onset is explosive with a sudden severe headache, nausea, vomiting, and some degree of loss of consciousness.
—Often caused by leaking or ruptured arterial aneurysm.
—Lumbar puncture will produce bloody (cerebrospinal fluid) CSF. Blood (or bacteria) in the subarachnoid space will cause nuchal rigidity.
—Patient should be kept quiet, in a dark room with minimal stimulation. Sedation, bedrest, and stool softeners are usually part of the therapeutic regime. Steroids may be given to try to reduce vasospasm.
—Blood in the subarachnoid space may obstruct the Aqueduct of Sylvius between the third and fourth ventricle or the channels exiting the fourth ventricle, which could result in hydrocephalus. The red cells in the CSF may also impair resorption of CSF, resulting also in hydrocephalus.
—If the subarachnoid hemorrhage is due to an aneurysm, an aminocaproic acid (Amicar) drip may be used to prevent further bleeding by blocking the normal lysis of the blood clot that has stopped the hemorrhage. The initial bleeding vessel is sealed by formation of a clot plus arterial spasm with dissolution of the clot after about 7 days. The chance for rebleeding is most likely to occur 7–10 days following the initial hemorrhage.

Differentiating bloody spinal fluid—SAH from traumatic spinal tap:
1. Blood will not clot in tubes if a SAH is present, but it will clot if blood is from a traumatic spinal tap.
2. All tubes of CSF are grossly bloody in presence of a SAH. Fluid will gradually clear in presence of a traumatic tap.

Primary Complications of SAH:
1. Hydrocephalus
2. Vasospasm
3. Dysrhythmias

Testing for a CSF Leak:
With bloody drainage from ear or nose use starch test—dab a small amount of drainage on a pillow case or other finely- woven material. If CSF is present the blood will migrate to the center of the spot, and there will be a clear halo ring around the blood. With clear drainage from ear or nose, use a glucose dipstick. If it is positive for glucose, CSF is probably present.

Coup and Contracoup Injury:
Coup injury involves damage to brain tissue directly beneath the area of impact.

Contracoup injury involves damage to brain tissue on the opposite side from the impact. This is a result of the brain banging against the inside of the skull on the opposite side from impact. Deceleration and acceleration are the two common mechanisms of injury causing a contracoup injury.

Hydrocephalus
Communicating hydrocephalus—nonobstructive. May be a result of a SAH which impairs reabsorption process of CSF, or an overproduction of CSF. The flow of CSF is normal.
Noncommunicating hydrocephalus—obstructive. There is an obstruction to the normal flow of CSF through the ventricular system.
Normal pressure hydrocephalus—a communicating hydrocephalus in which ICP remains normal despite an increase in CSF that causes enlargement of the ventricles. May be a result of head trauma, surgery, SAH, bacterial meningitis, or may be idiopathic.

Vasospasm:

The cause of vasospasm is not entirely clear. It usually occurs in the vessel adjacent to the ruptured aneurysm. Depending on its intensity, it may spread through the major vessels at the base of the brain, causing brain ischemia and possible infarction of brain tissue. Symptoms of vasospasm may occur after the initial bleed or postoperatively. Watch for hemiparesis, visual disturbance, seizures, or a decreasing level of consciousness!

Incidence of vasospasm is 30-50% preoperatively and 40-65% postoperatively. The site of the most common occurrence of vasospasm is with aneurysms in the internal carotid artery; the site of the least common occurrence is with aneurysms in the middle cerebral artery.

Theories of etiology and treatment of vasospasm:
1. One theory is that serotonin (a chemical produced in the GI tract and carried by platelets) is released from platelets following cerebral hemorrhage. Serotonin produces vasoconstriction and is a highly spasmogenic substance. Medications used are Reserpine and Kanamycin. Reserpine inhibits uptake of serotonin by platelets by exposing them to metabolic degeneration through cyclic monomine oxidase. Kanamycin sterilizes the GI tract, thereby ridding the bowel of the enzyme needed to produce serotonin.
2. The vascular smooth muscle constriction of vasospasm is thought to be relieved, according to a second theory, by an intravenous drip of sodium nitroprusside. If hypotension results, the drug can be slowed or stopped or a simultaneous infusion of dopamine can be used.
3. Isoproterenol increases levels of cyclic adenosine monophasphate (AMP) in vascular smooth muscle. Aminophylline works to inhibit the enzyme phosphodiesterase, which destroys cyclic AMP. It is thought that by increasing the levels of cyclic AMP within vascular smooth muscle, relaxation of the muscle will result by altering calcium binding and transport within the cell. So simultaneous infusion of isoproterenol and aminophylline is used.

—Rebleeding is the main cause of death in the unoperated patient.

Intracerebral Hemorrhage (Fig. 3.5)
—Occurs in 2% to 3% of head injuries.
—Hemorrhage is deep within the tissue of the brain, usually in a cerebral hemisphere.
—Main cause of intracerebral hemorrhage (ICH) is hypertension.
—There is a danger that a large clot will cause a shift of brain tissue and cause increased intracranial pressure.
—If patients can survive 7-14 days, then be operated on to remove the mass, they may wake up somewhat, and be a better candidate for rehabilitation.

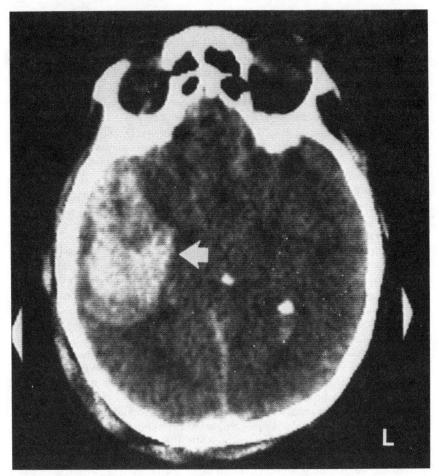

Figure 3.5. CT scan showing large right temporal intracerebral hematoma (*arrow*). (Reproduced with permission from Cooper PR (ed): *Head Injury*. Baltimore, Williams & Wilkins, 1982, p 223.)

Evacuation of the clot will not usually improve any focal deficits—that brain tissue is dead.

D. Skull Fractures

1. Linear Fracture—a break in the skull without displacement of the bone
—Constitutes about 70% of skull fractures.
—No treatment usually necessary unless vessels close to the skull are injured,

such as the middle meningeal artery, injury to which may cause an epidural hemorrhage.

2. **Depressed Fracture—a break in the skull causing inward displacement of the bone (Fig. 3.6).**
—Usually requires surgical elevation of the bone with debridement of bony fragments, if present.
—May cause laceration of surrounding brain tissue or meninges.
—Patient may require cranioplasty at a later date to replace section of the skull. Not done immediately after injury if increased intracranial pressure is expected. This allows room within the skull for swelling.

3. **Compound Fracture—a break in the skull causing a communication between the brain and the scalp.**
—Open communication increases risk of infection, often causing menigitis.
—Treatment involves debridement of the wound, closure of the track and use of antibiotics prophylactically.

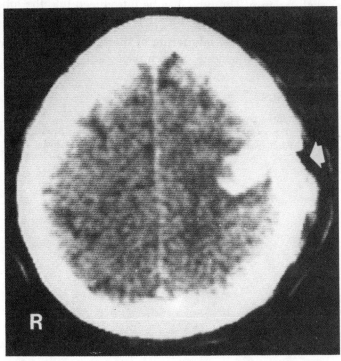

Figure 3.6. CT scan shows left-sided depressed skull fracture (arrow) and subjacent intraparenchymal hematoma. (Reproduced with permission from Cooper PR (ed): *Head Injury.* Baltimore, Williams & Wilkins, 1982, p 69.)

—May result in a CSF leak if dura is torn.

—Often involves nasal sinuses or tympanic membrane rupture.

4. Basilar Skull Fracture—a break in the skull at the base of the brain or involving the vault of the skull.

—Seventy-five percent of basilar fractures involve the petrous process of the temporal bone.

—Presence of otorrhea (drainage from the ear(s), rhinorrhea (drainage from the nose), or Battle signs [ecchymosis over the mastoid process behind the ear(s)] may indicate presence of a basilar skull fracture.

—Risk for infection is increased if CSF leak is present.

—Complications may include injury to the internal carotid artery as it enters the skull at the base of the brain, or venous sinuses, and cranial nerve injury.

—Bilateral or unilateral periorbital ecchymoses often present.

—Treated with bedrest, observation, and antibiotics if CSF leak is present.

—If CSF leak does not seal itself, surgical repair of the dural tear may be necessary. More likely to seal if the patient remains flat in bed.

—Caution must be taken when inserting a nasogastric tube into a patient with a basilar skull fracture. The tube may be introduced into the intracranial compartment.

5. Comminuted Fracture—a splintering of the skull into fragments.

—Craniectomy of bony fragments is often necessary.

SUGGESTED READINGS

Neurologic Disorders. Springhouse, Pa., Springhouse, 1984.
Pallett P, O'Brien M. *Textbook of Neurological Nursing,* Boston, Little, Brown, 1985.
Rudy E. *Advanced Neurological and Neurosurgical Nursing,* St. Louis, Mosby, 1984.

CHAPTER 4

Altered Levels of Consciousness

I. DEFINITION AND DISCUSSION

Consciousness is a state of awareness of oneself and the environment and the ability to respond to environmental stimuli. Consciousness consists of content (the ability of reasoning, thinking, and feeling) and arousal (referring to a state of wakefulness).

We usually visualize a reduced level of consciousness when there is discussion about an altered state or level of consciousness. This may not always be true, however. Delirium, confusion, and disorientation are often seen in patients following central nervous system dysfunction. These altered states of consciousness may be excitatory states.

Not all changes in level of consciousness are abnormal. Sleep is a normal altered state of consciousness. Dreaming and day-dreaming also are normal variations on the individual's baseline level of consciousness. Induction of anesthesia causes a temporarily altered level of consciousness that is not necessarily considered pathologic.

An individual's level of consciousness is very significant in patients with neurologic dysfunction. Clinically, it is the first parameter to change when a patient's neurologic status is deteriorating or improving. Any change from baseline may be significant. Very subtle clinical changes may be reflections of disastrous internal changes.

Nurses who care for patients with altered states of consciousness, especially the unconscious, face an unique challenge. The unconscious patient is unable to make his needs known, or verbalize internal clues, such as focal pain, feelings of nausea, dizziness, and double vision. The nurse is left to make the decisions about his comfort, safety, and other needs.

The cognitive-perceptual functional health pattern is often affected when an individual's level of consciousness changes. There may be disorientation to the environment, time, or person. The individual's attention span may be significantly shortened, so he is distractible and unable to consistently follow commands. There may be altered motor responses and perhaps no perception or response to external stimuli at all. Reflex responses to stimuli may be increased or decreased.

II. ETIOLOGY

1. General Information
Various terms are used to describe altered levels of consciousness.
—*Coma* is a state of unresponsiveness from which the individual cannot be aroused. There are areflexia and absence of awareness of self and the environment, even with stimulation. Coma is also defined as a Glasgow Coma Score of 7 or less. The word is derived from the Greek "koma," meaning lethargy or deep sleep.
—*Vegetative state, akinetic mutism,* or *coma vigil* are sometimes used interchangeably. They refer to a state in which sleep-awake cycles are present, but without evidence of cognition. The brainstem maintains internal homeostasis but there is no awareness.
—*Locked-in syndrome* is a state of consciousness in which there is evidence of mental functioning but there is no verbal or motor response because of selective deafferentation that causes paralysis of all extremities and the lower cranial nerves, but without loss of consciousness. Awareness of the environment may be demonstrated by eyeblinking on command.
—*Brain death* refers to a state in which all brain functions, including brainstem functions, are absent. Without an intact brainstem, even the vegetative functions such as heart beat, breathing, and blood pressure control, cannot be maintained very long.
—Stages of anesthesia:
   Stage I—involves the beginning of anesthesia to the loss of consciousness. Also referred to as the stage of analgesia, meaning that the sensation of pain is not lost, but the patient's response to the pain is altered.
   Stage II—(stage of delirium), includes the time between loss of consciousness to the onset of a regular breathing pattern and loss of the lid reflex.
   Stage III—includes the time between onset of a regular breathing pattern to the cessation of respiration. Most surgical procedures are done with the patient at some level of stage III.
      Plane 1—Lid reflex is lost and respirations are regular. Pupils are small. Eyes may oscillate.
      Plane 2—Pupils are fixed and eye oscillation stops. Tidal volume lessens and respiratory rate starts to increase.
      Plane 3—Intercostal paralysis results by the end of this plane, leaving diaphragmatic breathing.
      Plane 4—Pupils are dilated and fixed. Very little muscle tone is in evidence. Spontaneous respirations stop.

Stage IV—Includes the time from cessation of breathing to circulatory failure. Most reflexes are absent. This is a premortem stage.

2. Coma

There is a mnemonic which is helpful in recalling possible causes of coma:

A alcohol,
E epilepsy, encephalopathy (e.g., Wernicke's),
I   insulin,
O overdose (drugs, mediations),
U uremia,
T trauma,
I   infection,
P psychogenic condition,
S stroke, syncope.

Coma and other alterations in level of consciousness result from conditions which destroy or depress the reticular activating system (RAS) in the brainstem, or by diffuse dysfunction affecting both hemispheres. The RAS is thought to be responsible for our awake state. It consists of a system of neurons which receive nerve impulses from all sensory organs and from higher brain centers. Pathways from the RAS carry the incoming stimuli to the cortex and other parts of the brain. That continuous bombardment of the brain with stimuli keeps us in the awake state. Anything that interferes with the incoming stimulation to the brain via the RAS will also result in a less awake state. (Fig. 4.1)

Coma may result from the following four categories of dysfunction:

a. Supratentorial lesion. This is a hemispheric lesion which, due to its mass, presses on the brainstem, causing brainstem dysfunction. An example may be a subdural hematoma, a tumor, a hemorrhagic stroke, or an abscess.
b. Primary brainstem lesion with normal cerebral hemisphere function. Examples may be a brainstem stroke, abscess, or a cerebellar tumor.
c. Metabolic or diffuse disorders of the central nervous system at both the brainstem and hemisphere levels. These may include electrolyte disorders, drug or alcohol overdose, diabetic coma, anoxia, seizures, or encephalopathy.
d. Psychogenic states are rare, but may resemble coma, but have no discernable physiologic cause. Examples may be depression, conversion reaction, and catatonia.

3. PVS (persistent vegetative state)

Two to eight per cent of severe head injuries result in the persistent vegetative state. Severely brain-injured patients are being saved today with sophisticated technology that was not available even 10 years ago.

The PVS syndrome was first described by Jennett and Plum. They described the progressive behaviors of PVS as follows:

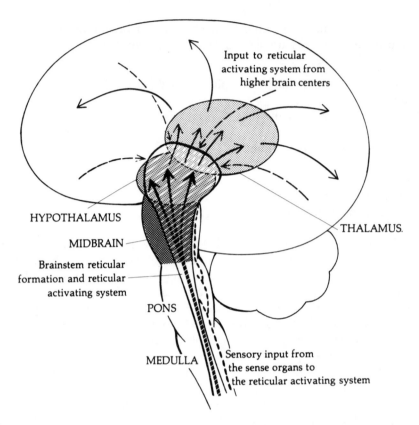

Figure 4.1. Diagram of the brainstem reticular formation and reticular activating system indicating afferent input to it from the organs of special sense and higher brain centers, and its action in arousal of the whole brain. (Reproduced with permission from Stephens G: *Pathophysiology for Health Practitioners*. New York, Macmillan, 1980, p 435.)

a. During the first week or so after injury patients are in deep coma. They do not open their eyes. When they react to stimulation, they usually demonstrate extensor (decerebrate) responses.

b. Within 2–3 weeks they usually begin to open their eyes, usually first in response to painful stimuli, and then to less noxious stimuli. The open eyes are inattentive. There is wakefulness without awareness. This suggests an intact RAS (reticular activating system) in the brainstem but a nonfunctioning cortex. Some coordinated motions, such as scratching, grasping, sucking, chewing, swallowing, and teeth-grinding may be present. Speechlessness is universally present. There may be frequent spells of excessive sympathetic nervous system activity.

c. The extensor (decerebrate) response may disappear after a few weeks, followed by flexor (simple) withdrawal response to painful stimulation.

d. Initially the patient may have a flat or isoelectric EEG, but activity may increase if the patient survives the PVS for several months.

Causes of PVS may be:

—Lesions in the cortex, subcortical structures of the hemispheres, the brainstem, or in all of these sites.

—Hypoxic or ischemic insults to the brain.

—Traumatic brain injury.

—Sequella to traumatic or nontraumatic coma.

4. Locked-in Syndrome

In this state the patient's face and extremities are totally paralyzed, but he is awake. He is unable to respond to stimuli. The cause is a lesion in the brainstem that damages the descending motor tracts to the face and extremities, but spares the RAS and innervation to the eyes. Eye blinking and vertical eye movements are the only voluntary functions possible. The reason for selective preservation of alertness and vertical eye movements is the preservation of the midbrain and pontine tegmental areas while the descending motor fibers in the pons are damaged.

The patient can be fully conscious of himself and the surroundings but he has been "locked into" a paralyzed body without a change in the level of consciousness. Alexander Dumas described a "corpse with living eyes" in *The Count of Monte Cristo*, and it is an appropriate description of a person with locked-in syndrome (LIS).

LIS is classified as follows:

a. Classic LIS usually results from a brainstem infarction, often due to basilar artery occlusion. The next most frequent cause is a hemorrhage in the pons varolii. Damage is thought to result from the mechanical stretching which occurs during hyperextension trauma. Heroin abuse has also been associated with LIS, presumably due to a hypersensitivity response.

b. Total LIS involves total immobility, including all eye movements. The only way to clinically distinguish this patient from the patient in coma is with EEG. The EEG of a patient with total LIS usually appears normal, and there is some correlation with the patterns associated with consciousness.

c. Incomplete LIS is a state where some motor function remains. There is often some weak arm or hand movement. Some movement of facial muscles, crying, or groaning have also been reported with incomplete LIS.

5. Brain Death

—Definition

For many years, death was thought to result when circulation stopped and vital functions such as respiration ceased. During the 1950s and 1960s cardiopulmonary resuscitation became common practice. Resuscitation teams soon learned that not everyone should be resuscitated. Patients who had prolonged periods of no respiration or circulation were not resuscitated because of recognition of the concept of brain death.

During the 1960s with the advent of organ transplantation, the medical community realized the need for a better definition of death. Since the report of the Harvard Ad Hoc Committee in 1968, there has been more widely acceptable consensus that patients who meet certain criteria for irreversible loss of brain function, are dead. The Harvard criteria for death conclude that the person is dead if the brain is dead. Most states currently have statutes that allow physicians to declare death on the basis of loss of brain functions.

—Criteria for brain death (Table 4.1)

Brain death is diagnosed when there is no evidence of either brainstem or hemisphere function for a prolonged period, usually 12 hours or more, and when the lack of brain function is the result of structural and not of reversible metabolic disease.

- Tests of cortical functioning

  Cerebral or cognitive functioning is tested by exposing the patient to stimuli such as light, sound, pain, and motion. In brain death, there is no response to verbalization, no spontaneous or coordinated eye movements, and an absence of motor response to pain. An EEG may be done to confirm brain death. Absence of intracranial blood flow may be documented with a brain flow study.

- Tests of brainstem functioning

  —There is no pupillary light reflex.

  —No eye movements are present with ice water calorics (oculovestibular reflex), and oculocephalic reflex is absent.

  —Vagus nerve functioning may be determined by injecting the patient with 0.1 mg of atropine. If the vagus is intact, the heart rate should increase by 5 beats per minute.

  —Because it is thought that the acoustic cranial nerve is one of the last portions of the brainstem to remain intact, brainstem auditory evoked responses can be tested. Absence of this response indicates widespread central nervous system damage, and is consistent with brain death.

  —Other cranial nerve functions which may be tested are the corneal reflex and gag reflex.

  —Spontaneous respirations are absent. The patient is disconnected from the ventilator for at least 3 minutes and the pCO_2 is allowed to rise to at least 55 mm Hg. Respiratory effort should be watched for (movement of chest, abdomen, neck, mouth) and possible air flow through the endotracheal tube should be felt and listened for.

6. Pathophysiologic Processes in Coma

—Coma may be associated with cerebral edema. Edema fluid is high in sodium and chloride content and also contain albumin. When this protein

Table 4.1.
Brain Death Criteria
(Adapted from the By-Laws of The New York Hospital)

Determination of brain death shall be made in accordance with the mandatory criteria listed below. All observations, tests and findings shall be recorded in the patient's chart. Supplementary criteria may be used at the physician's discretion.

Mandatory Criteria

I. Coma of established cause
   A. No potentially anesthetizing amounts of either toxins or therapeutic drugs can be present. Hypothermia below 30°C or other physiological abnormalities must be corrected to the extent medically possible.
   B. Irreversible structural disease or a known and irreversible endogenous metabolic cause due to organ failure must be present.
   C. A twelve-hour period of no brain function must have elapsed.
II. No cerebral function
   No behavioral or reflex response involving structures above the cervical spinal cord can be elicited by noxious stimuli delivered anywhere in the body.
III. No brainstem reflexes
   A. The pupils must be fixed to light.
   B. No corneal reflexes can be present.
   C. There must be no response to icewater caloric (50 ml in each ear).
   D. No spontaneous respirations must occur during apneic oxygenation for a period sufficient to maximally stimulate breathing.
NOTE: The circulation may be intact and purely spinal cord reflexes may be retained.

Supplementary Criteria

The twelve hour period of observation may be shortened to as little as 6 hours in cases of established irreversible structural damage provided that the mandatory clinical criteria are confirmed by one or more of the supplementary criteria.

I. An EEG for 30 minutes at maximal gain reflects absence of cerebral electrical activity.
II. Brainstem auditory evoked responses reflect absence of function in vital brainstem structures.
III. No cerebral circulation present on angiographic examination.

(These criteria are included with permission of the New York Hospital-Cornell Medical Center. Neither the author nor the hospital represents that these guidelines are or will continue to be acceptable under the laws of any particular state or will be applicable for every case.) (Reproduced with permission from Earnest, MP. *Neurologic emergencies.* New York, Churchill Livingstone, 1983, p 423.)

exudate is present, it implies a breakdown or leaking of the blood-brain barrier, thus homeostasis of the brain is compromised. Cerebral edema interferes with cerebral metabolism and may result in an increase in intracranial pressure (ICP). The blood flow to the brain is reduced when the ICP increases, and the brain may then become ischemic.

—Cerebral oxygen metabolism is usually impaired in patients with coma. The reason for the decreased metabolism is that damaged brain cells use less oxygen than normal cells.

The cerebral metabolic rate for oxygen ($CMRO_2$) is a method of determining how much brain injury is present. When the $CMRO_2$ is below 2.0, the patient is usually in coma.

—Glucose is the only organic nutrient able to cross the blood-brain barrier, thus it is the only normal substrate of cerebral metabolism. The brain does not store much glucose, and when the arterial levels fall to less than 20 mg/100 ml, coma results. Neuronal damage and death result from a glucose deficiency. When ischemia is present, as it often is in a patient in coma, there is stimulation of brain glycolytic activity, resulting in glucose depletion.

—Cerebral blood flow is affected by several physiologic changes. Lowered PO_2 causes an increase in cerebral blood flow (CBF): lowered PCO_2 decreases CBF; alkalosis decreases CBF. With a reduced CBF ischemic neurons may become anoxic, resulting in areas of brain tissue infarction. So patients in coma with ischemic areas of the brain may develop further damage of the brain, making coma a permanent state of consciousness.

—Neurotransmitters more recently have been thought to play a role in the state of consciousness. It is thought that catecholamine synthesis is affected when the brain receives an ischemic insult, thus aggravating brain dysfunction and causing neurotransmitter failure and cerebral infarction. Some postmortem studies of patients in coma or with brain infarction showed depletion of dopamine in all types of coma.

III. GENERAL TREATMENTS

A. Diagnostic Tests in Evaluating Levels of Consciousness

—The physical exam is vital in isolating a possible lesion causing the abnormal state of consciousness. For example, symmetry and nature of movements, pupillary size and reactivity, reflexes, and respiratory pattern are all important to note. Level of consciousness should be graded with the Glasgow Coma Scale.

—Computerized axial tomography (CAT scan).

—Magnetic resonance imaging (MRI) may be used.

—Lumbar puncture may be indicated once a space occupying lesion is ruled out.

—Toxicologic analysis is often used when the cause of coma or altered state of consciousness is unknown. Screening is usually done for ethanol, barbiturates, benzodiazepine, and narcotics. Some drugs, such as amphetamines and phenothiazines, are easier to detect in urine than in blood samples.

—Auditory brainstem responses (ABRs) help differentiate between central and peripheral nervous system pathology, and brain death determination.

—An EEG may be confirmatory in brain death determination and in diagnosing locked-in syndrome.

—A brain flow study documents presence or absence of blood flow to the brain, in determination of brain death.

—In differentiating a patient with a true neurologic deficit from the hysterical or malingering patient there are a few useful tips:

  • A malingerer wants either little examination or none at all. It is difficult to imitate a deficit. A hysterical patient may not mind being examined repeatedly, but the hemiparesis, numbness or other deficit may switch sides.

  • Some clues to the diagnosis of hysterical unconsciousness are that the patient is in a trance-like state. With his eyes open, he may alternate laughing and crying, be rigid and then move purposefully.

  • In hysterical coma, when the patient's eyelids are lifted he may focus on the examiner. The patient is showing resistence if the eyelids are forced open by the examiner and only the whites of the eyes can be seen (the eyes have reflexively rolled up in the head). A truely comatose patient's eyelids will close together when released, closing quickly at first, and then gradually. It is difficult to fake that gradual closing.

B. Medical Management

—Gastrostomy tube or jejunostomy tube insertion may be necessary for long-term feeding needs of a patient with a depressed level of consciousness. There is less likelihood of aspiration with these feeding tubes than with nasogastric tubes.

—Tracheostomy may be needed for adequate airway and secretion management.

—Treatment of increased intracranial pressure may be indicated (see Chapter 2) during the acute phase.

—Surgical intervention will depend on the specific cause of the altered state of consciousness.

C. Ethical Issues Surrounding Patients with Altered State of Consciousness

We currently have no accurate tool to predict outcome of patients in coma or various depressed states of consciousness. It may be very difficult to give a prognosis even several days after injury. Along with this limitation, we have an increasingly complex technology in the medical field. That allows us to keep patients alive longer than ever before. As technology increases, conflicts arise about the potential and actual application of this technology. Life can be extended quantitatively but not qualitatively. Without predictors of outcome, there seems to be a tendency to use a large amount of scarce resources on patients who may have little chance for recovery.

Society is becoming concerned about this issue of quality verses quantity of life. Legislative approval of living wills in many states may be a reflection of this societal concern. The public is asking questions such as, "Is it appropriate to spend hundreds of thousands of dollars on one heart transplant patient with uncertain outcome, or should that money go to provide proven, effective immunizations for all children?"

Where should our scarce resources be spent? The United States dialysis program adds $2 billion yearly to Medicare costs. Other countries have taken action to prevent such expense. England has legislated that dialysis is not available to patients over 55 years of age. China put all its dialysis equipment in a warehouse instead of choosing who got treatment and who did not. Future ethical decisions in the United States may revolve around who will be allowed to be treated, rather than when to stop medical treatment, which seems to be a current issue in this country.

Euthanasia is another issue being discussed a great deal. Killing and allowing to die are being debated. Hospices caring for terminally ill patients will not kill their patients, but they will allow them to die—by not treating pneumonia, for instance. The term comes form the Greek word, for good death, meaning death without suffering. The terms "active" and "passive" have been used to specify how death is produced. Active euthanasia usually refers to some positive, deliberate act(s) that are intended to cause death so a dying person would not suffer. It is viewed by practitioners as ethically unacceptable. It is also illegal in all the states. Passive euthanasia usually refers to a planned omission or a planned lack of interference with the death process. It is generally viewed as ethically and legally acceptable.

The President's Commission for the Study of Ethical Problems in Medicine and Biomedical and Behavioral Research decided that the acceptability of death by commission and death by omission should be based on other considerations as well. Health professionals often use the cause of death to assess the morality of an act or omission. Active and passive euthanasia end in the same result, death. Active euthanasia seems less acceptable because it is the act that may be viewed as the cause of death. With passive euthanasia, it is the underlying disease process that is viewed as the cause of death, rather than the omission.

Some authors view euthanasia as a death-oriented solution to the problem of how to care for the dying, since the resolution of the problem is death. They advocate that we focus more on enhancing the quality of the last phases of a dying patient's life.

Rationing of health care is a difficult concept for us in the health-delivery system to come to grips with, because we have never before had to consider it. There is a dynamic tension between cost containment and quality control. This is evident in issues around the DRG (diagnostic related groups) method of fiscal reimbursement to hospitals for care delivered. Putting a ceiling on the amount the hospital will be reimbursed for a specific patient condition engenders public fear that patients will not get the quality of care that is needed and may be discharged from the hospital too early. The DRG system makes physicians the fiscal agents for the hospital. Does that create a conflict of interest: what's the best for the patient verses what's best for the hospital? The physician's autonomy may be affected by the hospital's controlling his staff privileges to practice if he exceeds DRG payments. It seems appropriate that physicians should inform patients about cost constraints as a part of informed consent. This necessary rationing may have a strong impact on patients with uncertain or dubious outcome such as those in coma, PVS, or LIS.

Nurses have a role in the bioethical decision making process. In order to be knowledgable participants, nurses need to understand their own moral and ethical beliefs. Our own beliefs are tested very often when we care for patients in a vegetative state or in a coma. We ask "What is quality of life? Is human life defined as the ability to breathe? Breathe unassisted? Communicate? Think? Be happy?"

Jacques P. Thiroux in *Ethics: Theory and Practice*, (New York, Macmillan, 1986, p 404.) describes five principles to consider when making ethical decisions:

1. The reverence for life and acceptance of death. This means that life is important and is a basic right of all humans. Life is not everlasting, and "life at all costs" is not necessarily right. When a case is hopeless, extraordinary measures do not have to be used to maintain life. Right to life is a phrase used differently by different people. Does it include certain basics, such as nutrition?
2. Goodness or rightness. If an action produces pain, then it is not good, and if it produces disharmony, it is not right.
3. Justice or fairness. Humans should treat each other fairly and justly.
4. Trust and honesty. Communication should be based on truth.
5. Individual freedom. Each person has the right to decide his own destiny. A comatose patient may have made his wishes known with a living will.

Using these principles, we may begin to formulate our own beliefs.

The utilitarian theory of ethics stresses the consequences of action. It supports the least amount of harm or the most happiness for the greatest number of people. This seems to be in opposition to the medical ethic of saving everyone, regardless of cost. If we use this theory, we would approach ethical decisions by looking at the long-term effects to the individual, the family, and society. Acts of omission are seen as right or wrong in so far as they bring about an overall balance of good or bad consequences. Killing is wrong because it reduces happiness or promotes misery.

The human rights theory of ethics stresses doing no harm. Humans have rights that should not be violated. This approach does not accept that abuse of human rights can be justified by considering the overall good consequences. Acts of omission are seen as wrong only if there is a right to what has been omitted. Belief in the right to life would allow killing only when the right to life conflicted with the rights of others.

Predicting future suffering and discomfort associated with being comatose or in a vegetative or locked-in state is something a physician may be able to do. But deciding whether this suffering person would prefer to be dead is not a clinical decision. We cannot assume that death is preferable to a life of misery. Some people live lives of pain and suffering that we may think intolerable for ourselves. It may be very difficult to predict another's preference between these two conditions.

When a nursing unit is short of staff, which patient gets the least care? Is it the long-term comatose patient or the patient who has more potential for recovery? Do we feel guilty about making such an assignment? Do we ever say to ourselves, "What's the use of spending my time and effort on a patient who will never wake up?" Many of us have felt more discouraged than inspired when caring for a "hopeless" patient. We may wonder whether we are promoting the patient's life or simply prolonging his dying.

Some ways to cope with these feelings are, first of all, to recognize them. Establish rapport with the family and allow them to become involved in the patient's care. Involving the family may help them realize how much time and effort is required in caring for the patient. This may be useful if they are trying to decide whether they can take the patient home and care for him there. The care activities will also diminish the feelings of helplessness that families often have and help compensate for the lack of ability to communicate effectively with the patient.

Promote normalcy by talking to the patient and personalizing the room. This may help the patient, family, and the nursing staff. Pictures, for example, of the patient prior to injury may help us think of the patient more as an individual, even though we did not know him before hospitalization. In self defense, we may concentrate on the mechanics of treatment and not be concerned about the person we are treating. This may be more prevalent when we feel the patient is suffering.

Staff conferences or support groups may be helpful in verbalizing our feelings about caring for unconscious patients. Rotating assignments may be useful. Knowing we will only be caring for a particular patient for 2 to 3 days may allow us to provide a constant and high standard of care.

Ethical issues will not disappear, but may become even more complex in the future. Nurses need to become comfortable with their own beliefs so they can be useful in the decision-making process. As dimensions of nursing care expand, our role in this ethical decision-making process will also expand.

We hope some tool for predicting outcome from injury may be developed to help us make ethical decisions in a complex technology. Uncertainty of outcome at present leaves few alternatives but to presume that all patients have potential for recovery.

5

Cerebrovascular Disease

I. DEFINITION AND DISCUSSION

Cerebrovascular disease includes several different disease entities. It refers to a functional abnormality in the central nervous system caused by disease of the cerebral vessels. It may refer to occlusive disorders, such as a thrombotic or embolic stroke, or spasm of a cerebral artery. It may also refer to a hemorrhagic condition, such as a ruptured cerebral aneurysm or arterio-venous malformation (AVM).

Thrombotic and embolic strokes often involve the middle cerebral artery, which supplies blood and oxygen to the lateral side of the cerebral hemispheres. In-farction to that area may result in contralateral motor and sensory deficits.

—Cerebrovascular disease (CVD) is the most frequent neurologic disorder of adults.
—CVD is the third leading cause of morbidity and mortality in the United States, after heart disease and cancer.
—There are over 500,000 stroke cases (cerebrovascular accidents) in the United States every year. The number is declining, however. Only ⅓ of these stroke victims are able to return to a fully functioning life after stroke.
—Cyanotic heart disease is a common condition predisposing children to oc-clusion in cerebral vessels. Childhood infections and systemic diseases such as collagen diseases, intracranial hemorrhages, metabolic disorders, blood dyscrasias, and metastatic neoplasms are other frequent factors leading to stroke in childhood.

II. ETIOLOGY

—Thrombosis of a cerebral vessel
  • Often associated with atherosclerosis.

- Conditions such as sickle-cell disease and polycythemia may predispose a patient to thrombus formation. Infectious disorders and inflammation may result in cerebral thrombophlebitis.
—About ¾ of strokes are a result of obstruction (thrombus or embolus) of cerebral vasculature.
—Embolus in a cerebral vessel
- May be a result of a blood clot, fragments of an atheromatous plaque, lipids, or air.
- Emboli usually originate from the heart and go to the brain.
—Hemorrhage
- Hypertension usually is a precipitating factor. Cerebral aneurysms and arteriovenous malformations (AVMs) are more prone to rupture and cause a hemorrage in the presence of hypertension.
- Children with intracerebral or subarachnoid hemorrhage usually are not hypertensive, but the etiology more likely is trauma.
- Approximately ¼ of strokes are a result of hemorrhage.
- AVMs present most often in adulthood, especially between the ages of 20–40 years.

Pathophysiology of a stroke:
Oxygen deprivation of brain cells results from obstruction of cerebral vessels (thrombus or embolus). Oxygen deprivation causes loss of consciousness and hypoxic neurons, which become ischemic and eventually may become infarcted. At the point in time when the neurons are ischemic, there is a chance to reverse the ischemia and prevent infarction. This is an area of much recent research, trying to salvage ischemic areas and minimize the patient's deficits.

III. CLASSIFICATIONS AND CLINICAL MANIFESTATIONS:

—A patient may present with a transient ischemic attack (TIA) in which the neurologic deficit resolves within 24 hours. One-third of these patients will later have a major stroke.
—A patient may present with a reversible ischemic neurological deficit (RIND) in which the deficit remains beyond 24 hours, but eventually resolves completely.
—A patient may present with a completed stroke with a deficit that is permanent.
Definition of a stroke is:
- A focal neurologic deficit persisting longer than 24 hours.
- Sudden onset of the deficit.
- Vascular etiology (thrombotic or embolic occlusion of a cerebral artery resulting in infarction or spontaneous rupture of a vessel resulting in an intracerebral or subarachnoid hemorrhage).

Probable deficits of a left-hemisphere stroke:
—Right-sided hemiparesis or hemiplegia
—Right visual field defect
—Slow, cautious behavior
—Dysphasia

Probable deficits of a right-hemisphere stroke:
—Left-sided hemiparesis or hemiplegia
—Left visual field defect
—Spatial-perceptual deficits
—Poor judgment; impulsive behavior
—Distractability
—Unawareness of deficits of affected side

—Common clinical manifestations of a TIA, RIND, or a completed stroke include:
- Hemiplegia (on side of the body opposite the cerebral insult),
- Hemiparesis (on side of the body opposite the cerebral insult),
- Dysarthria (muscles for speech are impaired),
- Dysphagia (muscles for swallowing are impaired),
- Visual deficits such as double vision (diplopia), decreased visual acuity, or homonymous hemianopsia (loss of vision in the same side of each eye, contralateral to the lesion),
- Absent or diminished response to superficial sensation (touch, pain, pressure, heat, cold),
- Absent or diminished proprioception,
- Perceptual disturbances such as agnosia, apraxia, or disorientation to the environment,
- Dysphasia (Table 5.1)
  —Expressive dysphasia (Broca's) in which the patient is unable to produce understandable speech.
  —Receptive dysphasia (Wernicke's) in which the patient has no comprehension of the spoken word.
  —Global dysphasia in which the patient demonstrates both expressive and receptive deficits.
- Intellectual impairment, such as memory loss, poor judgment, inability to reason, calculate, and think abstractly,
- Emotional deficits, such as emotional lability, poor tolerance to stress, loss of self-control and social inhibitions, depression, withdrawal, confusion,
- Bladder and bowel dysfunction.

Other clinical manifestations of a leaking or ruptured AVM include:

Table 5.1.
Types of Dysphasia

	Expression	Verbal Comprehension	Repetition	Naming	Reading Comprehension	Writing	Lesion
Expressive (Broca's) Dysphasia	Nonfluent	Selectively intact	Impaired	Impaired	Variable	Impaired	Posterior-inferior frontal (Broca's area)
Receptive (Werniche's) Dysphasia	Fluent	Impaired	Impaired	Impaired	Impaired	Impaired	Posterior-superior temporal (Werniche's area)
Global Dysphasia	Nonfluent	Impaired	Impaired	Impaired	Variable Impaired	Impaired	Fronto-temporal

Reproduced with permission from Boss BJ: Dysphasia, dyspraxia, and dysarthria; distinguishing features, Part I. *J Neurosurg Nurs* 16(3):154, 1984.

Ninety-three per cent of the population is right-handed. This means their left hemisphere is dominant. Of the 7% of the population who are left-handed, about 60% have the dominant speech center in their left hemisphere also.

—Headache, often unilateral. It may be described as throbbing and synchronous with the heartbeat,
—Seizures, focal or generalized. Forty per cent of patients will have this as their first symptom,
—Paresis,
—Mental deterioration.

Pathophysiology of an AVM:
AVMs may be congenital defects. Some, it is thought, are acquired, as following a head injury when a shunt for blood develops around a clot. A clot in the dural sinus may also be a cause of AVMs, when revascularization occurs. There is a miscommunication among the arteries, veins, and capillaries. An AVM is a mass of arterial and venous channels with tortuous vessels of varying sizes. Blood is shunted through this network, and the arterial and venous supplies are mixed. AVMs often occur in the middle cerebral artery distribution, causing ischemia to surround cortical tissue. Arterial blood, which is shunted directly to the venous system, meets less resistance to flow than the normal capillary bed. Consequently the AVM receives a large blood flow. To handle this increased perfusion the arteries dilate, and to drain off the blood, the veins dilate.

An "intracerebral steal" refers to the pulling of blood flow away from one area of the brain as a result of the vascular resistance being lower in another area. AVMs may steal enough blood flow from another area of the brain to deprive that area of oxygen and glucose and cause ischemic changes to occur.

—Transient episodes of dizziness, syncope, confusion.
—Decreased vision.

Other clinical manifestations of a leaking or ruptured cerebral aneurysm include:

—Headache,
—Cranial nerve deficits,
—Lethargy,
—Meningeal signs (nuchal rigidity, photophobia, fever, irritability, positive Kernig's sign and Brudzinski's sign),
—Bruit (patient hears a noise in the head),
—Vomiting.

Pathophysiology of a cerebral aneurysm:

An aneurysm is an abnormal dilatation in the lumina of a cerebral vessel. Some are congenital malformations in the vessel wall, some may result from trauma, hypertension, or atherosclerosis. Most aneurysms (85%) occur around the anterior Circle of Willis, and most form at a point of artery bifurcation. Only about 15% of aneurysms occur within the vertebral-basilar system.

When aneurysms rupture they usually bleed into the subarachnoid space, although they may sometimes result in an intracerebral or subdural hemorrhage too. Types of aneurysms include:

—Berry aneurysms—have a stem and a neck.

—Saccular aneurysms—do not have a neck, but look like a bulging of the vessel wall. Ninety per cent of all aneurysms are berry or saccular.

—Fusiform atherosclerotic aneurysm—may become quite large, often on the basilar artery. May cause pressure on surrounding structures.

—Mycotic aneurysm—caused by an infected embolus or lesion of the arterial wall.

—Traumatic aneurysm—appears after traumatic head injury (blunt or penetrating injury).

IV. GENERAL TREATMENT

Diagnostic tests often used in CVD:

—CAT scan—helps differentiate vascular from nonvascular events in the brain. Areas of infarction may not show up on CAT scan for up to 48 hours.

—Arteriogram—demonstrates areas of possible carotid occlusion, arterial spasm, outline of an AVM or aneurysm, and abnormal blood flow patterns through the brain vasculature.

—Lumbar puncture—confirms suspicion of blood in the subarachnoid space.

—Brain scan—will make visible the areas of infarction, but not immediately.

A. Medical Management of Stroke

—Focus of treatment should be to salvage ischemic neurons which may be saved by providing oxygen, glucose, and blood flow.

• Provide adequate oxygenation.

• Provide nutrition to meet metabolic demands (patient is probably in a stress state).

• Maintain patient's cerebral perfusion pressure (CPP) at least at 60 mm Hg. Normal CPP is 80–90 mm Hg. Cerebral perfusion pressure is equal to the mean systemic arterial pressure minus the intracranial pressure (ICP). At a CPP of 40 mm Hg, cerebral blood flow begins to fail. At 30 mm Hg irreversible hypoxic changes leading to death occur.

• Mild hypertension is usually not treated. Lowering the blood pressure in a patient whose brain needs that high pressure to perfuse it, may cause major areas of infarction due to low CPP.

- Oversedation or rapid diuresis may precipitate a hypotensive episode, so should be avoided.
- Anticoagulation may be considered if stroke was due to a thrombosis or embolus.
- Increased ICP should be controlled (see chapter on Intracranial Pressure).

—Surgical intervention

- Endarterectomy may remove the thrombotic plaques occluding the artery, or may involve resecting a portion of stenosed artery. Often performed on the internal or common carotid artery.
- Extracranial-intracranial (EC-IC) bypass surgery is performed fairly frequently with some controversial results. The purpose is to increase blood flow to an area of the brain in order to prevent infarction. An extracranial vessel (usually the superior temporal artery) that perfuses the scalp is anastomosed to the middle cerebral artery (STA-MCA bypass). Thus collateral circulation is supplied to areas of the brain supplied by the middle cerebral artery. This procedure is sometimes done in patients with TIAs in hopes of preventing a future stroke.

    The overall operative mortality rate is approximately 3%. Fifty per cent of these deaths result from ischemic cerebral vascular accidents; the others are secondary to other postoperative complications such as subdural hematoma, intracerebral hemorrhage, septicemia, pulmonary embolus, and myocardial infarction.

—Patients with TIAs may be treated with antiplatelet drugs such as aspirin, persantine, or anturane. Making the platelets less sticky can help prevent a future stroke.

—Trental (Pentoxifylline) is an experimental drug being tested in the United States in treating chronic and acute obstructive arterial disease. Trental is thought to increase microcirculatory blood flow, thus improving perfusion and oxygenation to ischemic brain tissue.

—Experiments are being conducted in efforts to enhance the cerebral perfusion to ischemic areas by using Pentastarch (a plasma volume-expanding and hemodiluting agent). Lowering blood viscosity has been shown to elevate cerebral blood flow. Expanding plasma volume increases perfusion with a maximized cardiac output.

—Rehabilitation for motor and/or speech deficits should begin early.

B. Medical Management of AVM:

—Surgical resection of the AVM if it is accessible.
—Ligation of the arteries supplying the AVM. This is not possible when the arteries supplying the AVM also supply critical cortical areas.

—Embolization. Silastic beads are introduced into the internal carotid artery and enter the AVM. Thrombosis and destruction of the lesion results. A danger of the procedure is that dislodged a bead may migrate to the lung. Sometimes collateral circulation develops around the destroyed AVM, providing new blood supply and reactivating the lesion.

—The proton beam is a noninvasive treatment using radiation energy given off by protons accelerated in a cyclotron to shrink the AVM. It is available only in Berkeley, California and Boston, Massachusetts. It is useful for parenchymal AVM's deep within the brain or involving crucial areas such as those controlling motor function, speech, or vision. This method of treatment is new and somewhat controversial. It may take as long as 2 years for the effects of the treatment to occur.

—Propranolol hydrochloride (Inderal) may be used preoperatively and postoperatively to decrease the risk of postoperative hemorrhage. Cerebral blood flow can be 50 to 100% above normal with an AVM and cerebral autoregulation of blood flow may be disrupted. After removal of the AVM, increased blood flow is rerouted into the brain's normal circulation, which was accustomed to a reduced flow. Hyperperfusion results, and a hemorrhage may develop in the brain adjacent to the area of resection where most of the increased flow occurs. Propranolol is thought to decrease cerebral blood flow and cardiac output.

—Nd: YAG Laser (Neodynium: yttrium aluminum garnet) is a new treatment being tried with AVMs. Laser exposure is thought to coagulate thin-walled and fragile vessels. It causes a progressive contraction of the vessel wall, resulting in eventual closing of the vessel lumen.

C. Medical Management of Cerebral Aneurysms (Table 5.2)

—Subarachnoid hemorrhage precautions (see Chapter 3).

—Modify hypertension if present but maintain adequate CPP.

—Aminocaproic acid (Amicar) may be used to prevent fibrinolysis of the clot that has sealed the leaking vessel. Rebleeding and vasospasm are the major causes of death after the initial bleeding episode. Rebleeding is most likely to occur around the seventh day after the initial hemorrhage. Thirty percent of all patients rebleed within the two-week period after the initial insult. Two-thirds of these die from the rebleed.

—If hydrocephalus develops, a temporary ventricular catheter may be placed to drain off cerebrospinal fluid. If it is persistent, a permanent shunt may be surgically placed.

—If vasospasm occurs, there is no conclusive treatment. Increasing cerebral perfusion pressure by means of plasma volume expanders and pressor agents such as dopamine, seems to work to keep the vessels patent as well as any other treatment (see Chapter 3). Calcium channel blocking agents are being tested for their usefulness in treating vasospasm too.

Table 5.2.
Botterell Classification of Aneurysms

Grade	Criteria
Grade I (minimal bleed)	Patient alert, with no focal neurologic signs and no signs of meningeal irritation.
Grade II (mild bleed)	Patient alert with minimal deficits and usually signs of meningeal irritation.
Grade III (moderate bleed)	Patient lethargic, confused, with or without neurologic deficits and signs of meningeal irritation.
Grade IV (moderate to severe bleed)	Patient stuporous or comatose with some purposeful movements. Major neurologic deficits may or may not be evident.
Grade V (severe bleed)	Patient comatose and often decerebrate. Appears moribund.

—Surgical clipping and resection of the aneurysm may be performed. If resection is not an option, surgical plastic or gauze may be used to reinforce the walls of the aneurysm.

—Medications used with any acute cerebrovascular insult usually include those used to treat acute increased intracranial pressure (see Chapter 2).

CHAPTER 6

Seizures

I. DEFINITION AND DISCUSSION

A seizure is a sudden discharge of a group of neurons resulting in a transient impairment of consciousness, movement, sensation, or memory. It is not a specific disease process itself, but can be a manifestation of many different disorders.

—The term "epilepsy" is most often reserved to describe a chronic disorder involving recurrent seizures.
—The term "seizure disorder" may refer to either a recurrent condition or to one isolated occurrence.

    Epilepsy has had a negative connotation throughout history. It was once thought that evil spirits in a person caused him to have "fits." Insanity and mental retardation have also been linked with seizure disorders. Seizures, even today, are seen as a form of deviant behavior and may be frightening to the general public. The unpredictability and suddenness of the onset increase the fear.

Etiologies:

—Space-occupying lesions such as brain tumors or blood clots, uremia, metabolic disorders, overhydration.
—Trauma (5–50% of patients with head trauma develop posttraumatic seizures).
—Alcohol and drug overdose or withdrawal.
—Toxic substances such as heavy metals (lead or mercury).
—Meningitis or encephalitis.
—Electrolyte disorders.
—Cerebral anoxia.
—10–20% of patients with strokes develop seizures.
—Degenerative diseases such as multiple sclerosis, Alzheimer's, Pick's disease, or Huntington's chorea may be the cause of seizures.
—Hyperpyrexia in children.
—Some seizures may be idiopathic with no discernable cause.

II. CLASSIFICATION OF SEIZURES

International Classification of Seizures lists three different categories of seizures: partial, generalized, and unclassified.

Partial Seizures

Partial seizures involve abnormal electrical discharges from a focal area of the brain.

1. Simple partial seizures usually involve no impairment of consciousness. Symptoms include:
   —Motor (e.g. the Jacksonian March), clonic activity of any muscle group.
   —Somatosensory (e.g., tingling or numbness of a body part or visual, auditory, olfactory or taste sensations).
   —Autonomic symptoms (e.g., diapheresis, tachycardia, flushing).
   —Psychic symptoms are rare.
2. Complex partial seizures involve some impairment of consciousness. Focus for these seizures is often in or near the temporal lobe. Symptoms include
   —Cognitive disruption (e.g., deja vu or feelings of depersonalization).
   —Automatisms (e.g., lip smacking or playing with clothing).
   —Visual, auditory, or olfactory hallucinations that may cause bizarre behavior such as visualizing stars, hearing a voice tell them to do something, or smelling coffee brewing.
   —No recall of the behavior displayed; may be misdiagnosed as having a psychiatric disorder.

   Partial seizures may progress to become generalized seizures if the abnormal electrical impulses spread to involve the whole brain.

Generalized Seizures

Generalized seizures involve abnormal electrical discharges bilaterally within the brain. There are four types:

1. Absence seizures (petit mal): are most often seen in children and involve a transient loss of contact with the environment without violent muscular activity.
   —Typical absences and atypical absences differ primarily in the EEG pattern.
   —Atypical absences are often associated with mental retardation and some clinical automatism, such as lip smacking or chewing. Symptoms include:
   —Vacant staring, resembling daydreaming.
   —Minor motor involvement, such as eyeblinking.
2. Generalized tonic-clonic seizures (grand mal): start with the tonic or stif-

fening phase, followed by a clonic or jerking phase. Sometimes an individual has only one phase and not both. There is a postictal period (after the seizure) where the patient is exhausted and difficult to arouse. Symptoms include:

—Incontinence of stool and/or urine.

—Tongue-biting.

—Foaming at the mouth.

—Sudden loss of consciousness (always).

3. Generalized myoclonic seizures: these seizures may be present in patients with metabolic encephalopathies, degenerative diseases, or infectious processes. Symptoms include:

—A single jerk of one or more muscle groups, lasting only a second or two.

—No loss of consciousness.

4. Generalized atonic seizures: sometimes called a "drop attack" are often associated with myoclonic jerks. Symptoms include:

—Usually a loss of consciousness, but the event may be so brief that the patient is unaware he has had a blackout.

—Awareness of the attack comes with the sudden loss of muscle tone as he falls to the ground.

Unclassified Seizures

These are seizures (not in the above categories of the International Classification of Seizures) that either clinically or electrographically do not meet the established criteria, or the data available may be incomplete for diagnosis of the type of seizure.

Pseudoseizures

Pseudoseizures may closely resemble epileptic seizures, often making the diagnoisis very difficult.

—Occur most often in children and adolescents, affecting females twice as often as males.

—No abnormal electrical discharge from the brain with pseudoseizures. They are psychologically determined.

—Pseudoseizures usually occur in front of witnesses, and last longer than epileptic seizures.

—Patients may obey commands and demonstrate eye focusing during an episode.

—There may be environmental influences that affect or precipitate a pseudoseizure.

—Abnormal motor activity is present, but protective mechanisms remain intact, such as breaking a fall with arms or protecting head from hitting the ground.

—No tongue biting present, or incontinence or dilated pupils.
—Corneal reflex remains intact.
—Response to pain remains intact.
—Confusion after pseudoseizure is usually absent.
—Psychotherapy or hypnosis may be helpful intervention.

II. PATHOPHYSIOLOGY

The pathophysiology of seizures is not clear. Structural abnormalities in the brain have been implicated when found on autopsy of epileptic patients. However, these same structural abnormalities have been found in patients without a seizure disorder. When anatomic changes are found in the brain, research has not determined whether these changes are the cause or a result of the seizures.

Paroxysmal Depolarization Shift (PDS)

In a normal brain there exists a balance between excitatory and inhibitory synaptic influences on the postsynaptic neurons so that areas of excessive depolarization do not develp. When a seizure focus develops in the brain, the neurons become subjected to an abnormal or imbalanced pattern of electrical activity, called paroxysmal depolarization shifts (PDS).

—PDS may occur as a result of either excessive excitatory influences or insufficient inhibitory influences.
—When PDS develops, the electrical potential across the cell membrance delines toward threshold and, as this happens, numerous action potentials are generated in the neurons of the spike focus.
—Depolarization increases and persists and, as threshold is passed, there are no further action potentials but only extreme and prolonged electronegativity, which is recorded on EEG as the epileptogenic spike focus.
—Seizures begin at a specific focus but the wave of hyperexcitability may spread to other areas of the brain. The seizure may spread to normal neurons in the same anatomic area of the opposite hemisphere through connecting pathways, resulting in a mirror focus.

   Several theories for the cause of this mechanism have been developed, including the following three:

1. **Alterations of the Sodium Pump Mechanism**
   The sodium pump is responsible for maintaining the normal cell membrane resting potential. It does this by actively carrying sodium into the cell and pushing potassium out of the cell during depolarization. When neurons are deprived of the oxygen, glucose, or enzymes necessary for the active transport of sodium, there is a decrease in energy available. With no energy to keep the sodium pump functioning, sodium diffuses abnormally

into the cell and lowers resting membrane potential. When this happens neurons are more susceptible to rapid repetitive electrical discharges.

2. **Acetylcholine-Cholinesterase Imbalance**
Acetylcholine is an excitatory transmitter substance. It is necessary for normal impulse transmission across synapses. High levels of acetylcholine decrease the threshold for excitation of the resting membrane. This results in hyperactivity of the involved neurons. When cholinesterase is used up, the postsynaptic potential for inhibition is lost, resulting in a hyperexcitatroy state. If this excitation persists, it spreads to adjacent neurons, and results in a paroxysmal discharge of electrical activity.

3. **Alterations in the Conversion of Glutamic Acid to GABA (gamma aminobutyric acid)**
GABA is an inhibitory substance at the central synaptic level, and is produced by conversion of glutamic acid. Pyridoxine is the coenzyme that allows this conversion. When pyridoxine levels are low, GABA resources become depleted, creating a loss of inhibition and a hyperactive state in which repetitive firing of neurons results in a seizure.

How Seizures Stop

—Active inhibition by certain brain structures may end a seizure.
—Fatigue of the affected neurons may stop the tonic phase of a seizure, allowing muscles to relax.
—During the clonic phase, there may be intermittent recovery of the neurons for brief periods.
—Ultimately, the depletion of glucose and oxygen results in neuronal exhaustion, and the seizure stops.

III. GENERAL TREATMENT

The goal for medical management is to determine the underlying cause of the seizures and to treat it. Once the diagnostic tests are completed, management is determined. Diagnostic tests in the usual workup for a seizure disorder include:

A. Routine Laboratory Tests

—Blood chemistries:
  • Blood urea nitrogen (BUN).
  • Electrolyte levels.
  • Liver function tests.
  • Calcium and phosphorus levels.
  • Studies for toxic substances and alcohol (if history indicates).

- In children, blood and urine amino acid levels may help in diagnosing a metabolic etiology for the seizures.

B. Electroencephalogram (EEG)

This test is a physiologic recording, and does not distinguish one abnormality from another (that is, a tumor cannot be distinguished from a thrombosis by EEG). (See Chapter 1.)

—Recording the electrical activity in the brain may be useful in localizing the focus of onset of a seizure if it happens to be done when the patient is having a seizure.
—Many patients with seizure disorders have normal EEGs in the interictal phase. Ten per cent of patients with seizures have normal EEGs.
—There are various manipulation procedures that may be used during the EEG in an attempt to stimulate a seizure:
  - Hyperventilation.
  - Flashing lights.
  - Sleep or sleep deprivation prior to the EEG recording.
—Videotape monitoring of a patient concurrently with the EEG documents the clinical or behavioral component of the seizure activity shown on the EEG. Some patients can be monitored for 24 hours, thus documenting infrequent seizure activity that might otherwise be missed.

C. Lumbar Puncture

—A lumbar puncture (LP) is usually part of the diagnostic workup for seizures, unless contraindicated. (See Chapter 1, p 16.)
—Spinal fluid is analyzed for cell count, glucose, protein levels, and serology.
—Elevated opening pressure may indicate space occupying lesion (e.g. tumor). Signs of bleeding or infection may also be sources of seizure foci.

D. Skull X-Rays and/or Computerized Axial Tomography (CAT Scan)

—Skull films may reveal cranial growth asymmetry or intracranial calcifications. (See Chapter 1, p 13.)
—CAT scan allows visualization of anatomic structures inside the skull (tumors, infarctions, edema, hemorrhage, congenital lesions, and vascular abnormalities).

Medications

1. Anticonvulsants (Table 6.1)
Medical managment consists primarily of the use of anticonvulsant drugs to

prevent seizures by desensitizing the normal neurons to the barrage of electrical stimulation from the seizure focus.

—Approximately 70 to 80% of patients benefit from anticonvulsants.
—The drugs are chosen on the basis of the type of seizure disorder being treated since some drugs are quite specific in action.
—One drug is generally chosen to treat the seizure disorder and is given in increasingly higher doses until a therapeutic blood level is reached.
—If the patient continues to seize, a second drug may be started and given until it too reaches therapeutic blood levels.
—Different patients metabolize, absorb, and eliminate anticonvulsant drugs at different rates, so the dose required for different patients is individualized.

Surgical Intervention

The goal of surgical treatment is to remove the epileptogenic area with as little neurological deficit as possible.

—This is usually considered when the seizures cannot be controlled by drug therapy.
—Contraindications
  • Sometimes the seizure focus is in a part of the brain that is not accessible, and too much brain damage would be done in attempting to reach it surgically.
  • The surgical scar from the operation may be a future site for seizure activity; the patient may continue to have seizures even after surgery.
—Cerebellar stimulation is an experimental surgical procedure in which a brain pacemaker electrode is implanted in the cerebellum. A receiver is implanted in the chest, and may be pressed when the patient perceives an aura prior to seizing. This stops the seizure by sending inhibiting impulses to the cerebellum.

Status Epilepticus

Status epilepticus is said to exist when there are continuing or recurrent seizures in which recovery between attacks is incomplete. Clinical or EEG seizure activity which lasts 30 minutes or more is status epilepticus, and it is a medical emergency.

—Causes of status epilepticus in a patient with a known seizure disorder:
  • Noncompliance with the anticonvulsant therapy.
  • Subtherapeutic levels of the anticonvulsant due to a metabolic disorder.
—Causes in a patient without a known seizure disorder:
  • Head injury.
  • Subarachnoid hemorrhage.

Table 6.1.
Anticonvulsant Drugs

Drug	Nursing Intervention
For tonic-clonic seizures:	
Phenytoin (Dilantin)	Warn patient of possible side effects: –gastrointestinal upset –ataxia –nystagmus –diplopia –acne –hirsutism.
	Stress importance of good oral hygiene to minimize development of gingival hyperplasia.
	Warn about danger of suddenly stopping any anticonvulsant, as seizures may develop.
	Half-life is 24 hours, so may be taken once a day.
	Phenytoin increases metabolism of digitalis or warfarin.
	Causes discoloration of urine (pink, red or brown).
	When giving i.v. in hospitalized patients, use cardiac monitor and watch for widening of QRS complex and bradycardia. Give only 40 mg/min. Rapid infusion may also cause hypotension and cardiac arrest. Give in normal saline or lactated Ringers, as it will precipitate in dextrose.
Phenobarbital (Luminal)	Warn patient of possible drowsiness which may be dangerous if driving.
	Long half-life, so may be taken once a day. If taken at bedtime, some of the drowsiness is eliminated.
	Report the following to physician: –dizziness –fever –rash –nystagmus –irritability

Table 6.1.
(Continued)

Drug	Nursing Intervention
	–loss of libido –confusion in elderly –hyperactivity in children.
	Increases metabolism of digitalis.
	Decreases warfarin absorption.
	Potentiated by valproic acid.
	Potentiates phenothiazines.
	Tolerance may develop.
	i.v. administration may cause respiratory depression or arrest.
Primidone (Mysoline)	Similar side effects as phenobarbital, since it contains phenobarbital. Also may cause diplopia.
	Potentiated by isoniazid.
	Coumarin and ethanol affect metabolism.
Carbamazepine (Tegretol)	Half-life is short, so must be taken every 8 hours.
	Warn patient of possible side effects: –dry mouth –nausea, vomiting –drowsiness –ataxia –dizziness –jaundice –edema –rash.
	Decreases phenytoin levels.
	May cause inappropriate secretion of antidiuretic hormone in toxic levels, so have patient report reduction in urine volume.
	Use with caution if patient has glaucoma. Conjunctivitis and other eye changes, such as lens opacities, have been reported.
Mephenytoin (Mesantoin)	Warn of same side effects as phenytoin.

(continued)

Table 6.1.
(Continued)

Drug	Nursing Intervention

For absence attacks:

Ethosuxamine (Zarontin)

Warn patient of possible
-gastric upset, which may be minimized by
 taking it with meals
-drowsiness
-dizziness
-headache
-hiccups
-loss of appetite
-euphoria
-irritability
-urinary frequency
-swelling of tongue.

Methsuximide (Celontin)

Warn patient of same side effects as
ethosuximide plus:
-diplopia
-ataxia
-depression.

Trimethadione (Tridione)

Warn patient of possible:
-gastric upset
-drowsiness
-hiccups
-dizziness
-diplopia
-photophobia.

Valproic acid (Depakene)

Warn patient of possible:
-nausea and vomiting, which may be
reduced by taking it with meals
-drowsiness
-ataxia
-transient hair loss
-diarrhea and stomach cramps when toxic
levels are reached.

For complex partial seizures:

Phenytoin (Dilantin)
Phenobarbital (Luminal)
Primidone (Mysoline)
Mephenytoin (Mesantoin)
Carbamazepine (Tegretol)

Table 6.1.
(Continued)

Drug	Nursing Intervention
Phenacemide (Phenurone) Trimethadione (Tridione) Quinacrine (Atabrine) Clonazepam (Clonopin)	
For status epilepticus:	
Diazepam (Valium)	May be given i.v. to quickly stop a seizure, especially important if patient is having respiratory difficulty.
	Give in conjunction with an anticonvulsant, so by the time it starts to lose its effect, (half-life is short), the anticonvulsant is beginning to take effect.
	Watch for respiratory depression with i.v. use.

- Intracerebral hemorrhage.
- Encephalitis, meningitis.
- Hypoglycemia, hyponatremia.
- Acute alcohol or drug withdrawal.
A. Convulsive status epilepticus may include tonic-clonic muscle activity or muscle twitching. It is the easiest clinically to detect and is the most common type. There is also absence status, where clinically no violent muscle activity is seen, but confusion and inattention may be seen.
B. Focal status involves a repetitive clonic-type movement, usually of the face or arms. Electrical status may be seen on EEG with little or no clinical evidence of seizure activity. It may be suspected postoperatively when a patient with a craniotomy does not wake up as expected.

IV. NURSING MANAGEMENT

Nursing intervention is different when the patient is actively seizing than when he is over the acute phase and is ready for education about the disorder. The role of the nurse is vital in both stages.

A seizure disorder may be anxiety provoking for a patient and his family and friends. For the patient, the diagnosis of seizures may conjure up great fear of being out of control. There may be embarrassment at being a spectacle in public, including being incontinent in public. When amnesia occurs around the seizure event, anxiety may appear.

Restrictions placed on a patient with seizures, (for example, inability to drive a car, and having to take medication faithfully), are burdens. During different times in our life these restrictions may have different impacts. For instance, the inability to drive a car for a teenager may have widespread implications on his social life and peer associations, but the actual inconvenience may be minor. A traveling salesman in his 40s who is suddenly told he cannot drive will experience severe inconvenience and an impact on his livelihood.

Seizure patients may be feared by family and friends, as well as by the public in general. Some of this fear is due to the unpredictability of the occurrence and lack of knowledge about what to do if someone does seize in public. Neuro patients in general, and patients with seizures specifically, are often viewed with hesitancy by the public. People may fear the patient is mentally unstable, instead of viewing the deficit as simply a physical alteration.

A. Acute Phase

A witness to a patient having a seizure can be a valuable source of help with the history, for the patient often will have no memory of events just before and during the seizure. If a nurse is a witness to a seizure, there are several observations which should be made.

1. Onset
Note the time of onset of the seizure activity. Was it a sudden onset, or was it preceded by a warning aura? Was there an epileptic cry just before the onset?

2. Duration
Time the duration of the seizure from onset to completion.

3. Motor Activity
Observe the parts of the body involved and the order of involvement, and the character of the movements. Was the motor involvement symmetrical or was it unilateral? What was the first part of the body to demonstrate the seizure activity?

4. Eyes, Tongue, Teeth
Note eye or tongue deviation to one side or turning of the head. Check pupils for size and reactivity. Is nystagmus present? Were the teeth clenched or open?

5. Level of Consciousness
Check the patient for arousability during and after the seizure. If nonarousable, what was the length of that phase? Upon being arousable was the patient confused or fully aware? Was there memory for the event? Generally patients do not respond to their environment during a seizure, such as when their

name is called or when asked to follow commands. Sometimes patients trying to fake a seizure will respond during the seizure.

6. Respirations
Observe the rate, quality, pattern, or absence of respirations. Watch for cyanosis.

7. Body Activities
Report incontinence (urinary or fecal), vomiting, foaming at the mouth, bleeding from the mouth or tongue.

8. Postictal State
Note if the patient complains of numbness, weakness, tingling, muscle soreness, transient hemiplegia (Todd's paralysis). Were the motor alterations symmetrical or unilateral? Was aphasia present after the seizure? Was amnesia present? Were there other bodily injuries, such as from hitting the head or falling?

9. Precipitating Factors
Conversation with the patient may bring to light some precipitating factors, such as fever, emotional or physical stress, anticonvulsant noncompliance, or lack of sleep.

Seizure flow sheets may be a useful tool to collect and document all the observations made on a hospitalized patient. One example is shown in Figure 6.1.

If a nurse comes upon a person who is seizing, it is important to protect him from the environment. Airway maintenance is crucial. If the patient already has his teeth clenched, a tongue blade or oral airway should not be introduced. Usually teeth will only be broken and perhaps aspirated. Tongue blades or airways are helpful only if introduced before the teeth become clenched.

The patient should be rolled on his/her side to avoid aspiration if vomiting should occur. Restrictive clothing around the neck should be loosened to facilitate breathing. If possible, privacy should be provided for the patient. Restraining the patient should not be attempted. Reorienting the patient following the seizure may be reassuring to a person who is often very frightened when finally aware of what has happened.

If the victim of the seizure is in an inpatient hospital environment, bedrails should be padded and the bed left in the low position. If an aura precedes the seizure, the nurse may teach the patient to call for help and lie down wherever he is when the aura first occurs. This may prevent a fall and other injuries.

Rhabdomyolysis or myoglobinuria is a fairly common complication seen in hospitalized patients following seizure activity. It is often an alert nurse who notices the first signs of it, so prompt intervention can be initiated. Myoglobin is an iron-containing pigment found in skeletal muscle, especially

SEIZURE ACTIVITY SHEET

Patient's Name _____

Room No. _____ Age _____

Physician _____

Date	Time	Before			During								After				
		Warning Signs	Part of Body Where Seizure Began	General or Localized	Type of Movement	Duration of each Phase		Level of Conscious-ness	Pupils	Other		Behav-ior	Paral-ysis	Loca-tion of Paral-ysis	Sleep	Nurse's Initials
						Tonic	Clonic									

Figure 6.1. An example of a seizure activity chart. (Reproduced with permission from Hickey J: *The Clinical Practice of Neurological and Neurosurgical Nursing.* Philadelphia, Lippincott, 1981, p 459.)

in those specialized for sustained contraction. Seizure activity causes muscle damage. Severe exercise, such as military calisthenics, marathon running, jogging, riding mechanical bulls can all cause the same type of muscle breakdown. Patients with heroin or amphetamine overdoses (with the accompanying shaking chills) and those with phencyclidine (PCP, angel dust) abuse, where there is unusual muscular hyperactivity, or patients found lying unconscious for a period of time all may develop severe rhabdomyolysis.

The protein from the destroyed tissue causes the patient's urine to turn red or cola colored. The muscle cell breakdown releases myoglobin into the bloodstream, which is rapidly filtered by the kidneys, producing the dark urine. The myoglobin can occlude the kidneys and cause renal failure.

Treatment of rhabdomyolysis is to flush the kidneys. Furosemide and/or Mannitol may be used to help with diuresis, along with volume replacement. The hyperkalemia due to the cellular breakdown and renal dysfunction may also require treatment.

B. Long-term Phase

Once the diagnosis of seizure disorder is made, the most common therapy is the use of anticonvulsants. The nurse can do much in the way of patient education about the drug or drugs prescribed by the physician. The importance of taking the drug should be stressed, as well as possible side effects. Common side effects of many anticonvulsants include central nervous system (CNS) symptoms such as mental dullness, drowsiness, ataxia, and diplopia. Nausea, rash, gingival hyperplasia, an increase in body hair, and thickening of facial features may also be present. Some of these symptoms may be alleviated by having the patient aware enough of them to report them to the physician or nurse, so the dosage may be adjusted.

Patient referrals to national organizations, such as the Epilepsy Foundation of America, may be helpful as further information or education sources. Some of the national organizations also provide group insurance, vocational and employment programs, and low-cost prescriptions.

Situations that may precipitate a seizure should be discussed with the patient and family, so they can try to avoid them. Education about what to do in case of a seizure is also important. Patients as well as families can demonstrate great fright about seizures, especially the unexpectedness and unpredictability of occurance. If they are armed with knowledge about what to do in case a seizure occurs, often some of the fear is removed.

The patient should be encouraged to wear a Medic Alert bracelet or necklace that indicates the medical problem, the physician's name and phone number, and the medication the patient takes. Regular medical followup and evaluation should be encouraged.

As a result of interacting with the patient and family, the nurse can often get a feel of how they will be able to cope with the fact that a family member has a seizure disorder. If the coping skills seem minimal, perhaps psychiatric and/or social worker intervention is appropriate.

Family members, especially parents, often carry feelings of guilt about the seizure disorder. This can result in overprotectiveness and prevent the individual from developing independently. At the other extreme, the person with the disorder may become the scapegoat for the family, and all the family troubles may be attributed to this one person.

Social isolation is a problem which may be internally or externally imposed on a person with a seizure disorder. All efforts should be made to encourage the family and the patient to live as normal a life as possible despite the invisible disability. Society's sensitivity to the problem of seizure disorders is increasing through public education, and we hope it will continue to increase. It can have a significant influence on how an individual learns to cope with this disorder.

SUGGESTED READINGS

Earnest M: *Neurologic Emergencies*. New York, Churchill Livingstone, 1983.

Hickey J: *The Clinical Practice of Neurological and Neurosurgical Nursing*. Philadelphia, Lippincott, 1981.

Rudy E: *Advanced Neurological and Neurosurgical Nursing*. St. Louis, Mosby, 1984.

Snyder M: *A Guide to Neurological and Neurosurgical Nursing*. New York, Wiley, 1983.

Stephens G: *Pathophysiology for Health Practitioners*. New York, Macmillan, 1980.

CHAPTER **7**

Spinal Cord Injuries

I. DEFINITION AND DISCUSSION

An injury to the spinal cord can potentially affect every system of the body. It can be a catastrophic injury that changes a person's life completely. The incidence of spinal injury may be considered low in comparison to some other types of neurologic injury or disease, but the cost—both monetary and emotional—is high.

The incidence of spinal cord injury in the United States is approximately 10,000 each year, 7,000 to 8,000 of which survive and become paraplegics or quadriplegics. There are currently about 150,000 people with spinal injury in this country. Approximately 82% of spinal cord injuries involve young males (mean age of onset for all spinal cord injuries is 28.7 years).

Estimates of the lifetime costs for care of a quadriplegic are $325,000 to $400,000, and for a paraplegic $180,000 to $225,000. These costs are a burden on the injured individual, the family, and often, eventually, on society. Fifty-three to 57% of all spinal cord injuries result in quadriplegia.

The alteration in physical mobility is one of the primary nursing diagnoses applicable to the patients with spinal cord injuries. Mobility is the ability to move around freely without assistance. It denotes independence. Control over one's body is often taken for granted until it is suddenly lost. There is often some degree of paralysis or paresis following spinal cord injury. The impaired physical mobility certainly affects the activity-exercise functional health pattern of the individual. Mobility may be partially reinstated with artificial devices, such as a wheelchair or leg braces, but the patient's own body mobility is usually permanently impaired.

American society views physical vigor as a prerequisite for success. Television stars and athletes bring this view to youngsters. There is often a stigma attached to a person with a disability, evidenced by the difficulty reported by the disabled in getting jobs, establishing long-term relationships, and even getting access to many public places. This societal view is a difficult one to overcome and change.

II. ETIOLOGY

—The most common causes of spinal cord injury (SCI) are:
- Auto accidents (38%).
- Falls or jumps (16%).
- Gunshot wounds (13%).
- Diving accidents (9%).
- Motorcycle accidents (7%).

—These causes suggest that preinjury personality characteristics may be a contributing factor to spinal cord injury. There is disagreement among professionals in the rehabilitation field over the role of premorbid personality factors as related to risk behavior and incidence of traumatic injury. It is thought, however, that a person with high ego strength and the ability to delay gratification before injury will be better able to cope with sudden disability. Highly ambitious persons adapt less well.

III. CLASSIFICATION

A. Cervical Spinal Cord Injury

—Involves cervical region of the cord.
—May result in quadriplegia (tetraplegia) or quadriparesis with accompanying sensory impairment.
—May result in impaired respiratory function and impaired sympathetic system which innervates blood pressure, heart action, and body temperature.
—The cervical vertebrae have the greatest mobility and are quite unstable when subjected to trauma.
—The most common site of cervical body fractures is C5.
—The most common site of fracture dislocation is C5–C6.

B. Thoracic Spinal Cord Injury

—Involves thoracic region of the cord.
—Complete injuries below the T1 segment of the cord paralyze the lower extremities and impair trunk control to different degrees. This is paraplegia.
—The thoracic vertebral column is stabilized by the ribs.

C. Lumbar Spinal Cord Injury

—Involves lumbar area of the spinal cord.
—The heavy lumbar vertebrae are supported by large lumbar paraspinal muscles. These vertebrae have more stability than the cervical region, but less than the thoracic region.
—The conus (the tip of the spinal cord) is located at L1 and contains the micturition center for bladder control.

—Second most common site of injury to the spinal cord is in the lumbar region.

IV. PATHOLOGY

A. Mechanisms of Injury

1. Flexion-Rotation, Dislocation, or Fracture Dislocation Injury

—This type of injury usually occurs in the cervical region, particulary at C5–C6.

—Usually one or both posterior facets become subluxated or dislocated and locked. Nerve root compression may also result.

—Rotation may cause vascular damage, resulting in ischemia to the spinal cord.

—Traumatic flexion may cause a wedge compression fracture of the vertebral body, with a dislocation. The spinal canal becomes narrowed due to the malalignment.

—Most thoracolumbar spine injuries are of the flexion- rotation or fracture dislocation type.

—Most thoracolumbar injuries occur at the T12–L1 level.

2. Hyperextension Injury

—Most common in older patients with degenerative changes in the spine.

—Often follows stretching of the spinal cord against the ligamenta flava of the vertebral bodies. This may contuse the dorsal column of the cord and dislocate the vertebrae posteriorly.

—Often results in complete transection of the cord.

3. Compression Injury

—The lumbar and lower thoracic vertebrae are commonly compressed from the force of impact.

—The impact may cause the vertebral body to burst and bone fragments and disk material may be forced back into the spinal canal.

—In the cervical region C5–C6 is the most common level for this injury to occur.

—Only about half these injuries result in a complete neurologic deficit below the level of the injury.

B. Degree of Injury

—Complete spinal cord injuries are those in which no nerve fibers are functional distal to the level of the injury. It results in permanent loss of motor and sensory function below the level of the lesion. This patient will closely follow the dermatome chart for level of sensation.

—Incomplete spinal cord injuries are those in which some nerve fibers are preserved distal to the point of injury. This patient may vary somewhat from the dermatome chart for level of sensation. The prognosis is better in a patient with an incomplete injury, since he will be able to perform more motor activities and have more sensation than a patient with a complete injury, even though the levels of injury are identical.

A common test to determine if the spinal cord injury is complete or incomplete is the bulbocavernosus reflex. A rectal exam is performed and the glans or base of the penis is pinched or the examiner tugs on the Foley catheter. Involuntary contraction of the rectal sphincter during this maneuver indicates a positive reflex. This indicates that there is no physiological connection between the lower spinal cord and the supraspinal centers, and is a characteristic of a complete injury. Voluntary contraction of the sphincter or rectal sensation implies continuity of the supraspinal centers and prognosis of further motor and sensory recovery is probable.

C. Level of Injury

—Functional levels are very important in a patient with a spinal cord injury. Naturally we would like the patient to have the maximal functional ability possible. So the descriptive label we give a patient should reflect the functional level. The orthopedic level of injury may be different from the functional level, and it is really not significant in terms of what that patient will be able to do. For instance, the orthopedic level of injury may be a fracture at the C5 level. The nerves, however, may be intact to C6. So the patient is a C6 quadriplegic, not a C5.

D. Functional Levels

—The higher the injury is on the spinal cord, the greater the loss of motor activity and sensation.
—With a C1–C4 lesion, the intercostal muscles and often the diaphragm are paralyzed and there is no voluntary movement below the level of the injury. Sensory loss for the levels C1 through C3 include the occipital region, the ears, and some regions of the face.

Patients with a C1, C2, or C3 quadriplegia require a full-time attendant because they are dependent on a mechanical ventilator. They need assistance for all activities of daily living (ADL) such as bathing, feeding, and dressing. They can operate an electric wheelchair.
—A C4 quadriplegic also usually needs mechanical ventilation, but it may be used intermittently instead of continuously. He still needs assistance with ADL, but a feeding device may be adapted to his hand so that he can feed himself.
—A C5 injury spares the diaphragm, although in the acute phase, mechanical ventilation may be necessary due to ascending swelling around the cord. The C5 quadriplegic is dependent for most ADL, but may feed himself

with assistive devices, as well as write and dress his upper extremities. Wheelchair transfers are not independent.

—With a C6 lesion, a patient can do most of his ADL independently. He can feed himself without mechanical devices. He is able to drive a car with hand controls. There is loss of elbow extension and some hand function.

—There is potential for independent living with a C7 injury. Transfers are independent. Loss of sensation extends up the trunk to the level of the axillae and involves the inner arms and forearms and the ulnar area of the hands, including the fifth, fourth, and third fingers.

—A C8 quadriplegic may also live independently without attendant care. A sitting position can be supported well at this level.

—T1 to T5 paraplegics may have diaphragmatic breathing because of impairment of the intercostal muscles.

—From the level of T6 and below, there is usually spastic paralysis in the legs. Injury at T6 abolishes all abdominal reflexes.

—Injuries of L1 to L5 are independent in motor abilities but sensation is impaired in the legs and saddle region.

—S1 through S5 injuries may result in some displacement of the foot. There is no paralysis of the legs with S3 through S5 injuries. Sensation is impaired around the saddle area, scrotum, glans penis, perineum, upper third of the posterior thigh, and anal area.

E. Anatomical Level of Injury

—Neurons composing the descending pathways from the brain to the spinal cord are upper motor neurons (UMN). Injury to upper motor neurons can occur only above the L1–L2 vertebral level, since that is where the cord ends, and all upper motor neurons begin and end within the central nervous system.

—UMN injuries result in muscle spasticity and increased tendon reflexes.

—A lower motor neuron (LMN) injury occurs in the anterior horn cells or somewhere along the nerve fiber after it leaves the spinal cord. LMNs originate in the anterior horn cells of the cord and end in the muscle fibers.

—LMN injuries result in muscle flaccidity, loss of muscle tone, muscle atrophy, and loss of reflexes.

F. Spinal Shock

—The cause of spinal shock is thought to be the sudden loss of impulses from the descending pathways, which normallly maintain the cord neurons in a ready state of excitability. The absence of facilitation or excitation disrupts transmission at the synapse and impairs or prevents conduction of impulses. So the cord is unable to respond for a period of time.

—Spinal shock may occur 30–60 minutes after inury, and some aspects of it may last for months.

—Characteristics of spinal shock include:
  • Flaccid paralysis below the level of injury.
  • Absence of all cutaneous and proprioceptive sensation.
  • Hypotension and bradycardia.
  • Absence of reflex activity below the level of injury. This may cause urinary retention, bowel paralysis, and ileus. There is also loss of temperature control. The body tends to take on the temperature of the environment. Vasoconstriction and inability to shiver make it difficult for the patient to conserve heat in a cold environment, and the inability to perspire prevents normal cooling in a hot environment.

—Reappearance of a reflex that has been depressed after injury is a sign that spinal shock is resolving. The phases of recovery include:
  • Evidence of minimal reflex activity (usually within 3–6 weeks).
  • Evidence of flexor spasms in paralyzed limbs (usually within 6–16 weeks).
  • Alternation of flexor and extensor spasms in the paralyzed limbs (usually within 4 months).
  • Evidence of mainly extensor spasms (usually within 6 months).

—Usually, reflex acitivity returns in segments farthest from the level of cord injury first. Reflex activity is usually hyperactive, since it is without the inhibiting influence of the cortex.

—Reflexes do not return with an LMN paralysis. The flaccidity is permanent.

G. Autonomic Dysreflexia

—Autonomic dysreflexia is a syndrome that is a medical emergency. The symptoms are a reflection of an excessive autonomic response to a stimulus in patients with a cervical or high thoracic lesion, usually at T6 or above. The symptoms include:
  • Paroxysmal hypertension.
  • Pounding headache.
  • Blurred vision.
  • Profuse sweating above the level of the injury.
  • Flushing or splotching of the face and neck.
  • Piloerection.
  • Nasal congestion.
  • Bradycardia.
  • Nausea.
  • Pupil dilatation.

—Precipitating factors may be:
  • Bladder distention is the most common cause of autonomic dysreflexia. It

may also be caused by too rapid a decompression of a full bladder or by bladder spasms.
- Distended or impacted bowel or stimulation of the rectal mucosa while the patient is performing his bowel program (during digital stimulation or evacuation of feces).
- Pressure sores or skin stimulation. Decubiti and ingrown toenails are common stimuli. Any infection below the level of the lesion may initiate the reaction.
- Sexual activity. Ejaculation by a man.
- Uterine contractions during labor.
- Menstrual cramps.
- Intraabdominal irritation from disorders of the viscera.
- Spasticity.
- Tight clothing.
- Exposure to hot or cold stimuli.

—Physiological mechanism:
- Sensory receptors are stimulated at the offending site (bladder, bowel, skin). Impulses are carried by the spinothalamic tracts and the posterior columns. Because of the spinal cord lesion, the impulses do not reach the centers in the brain for interpretation of the stimulus. As the impulses go up through the lower cord stump, they activate a sympathetic reflex which produces the symptoms of autonomic dysreflexia. In a person whose cord was intact, the sympathetic reflex would be inhibited by an outflow of impulses from the brain. But with a spinal cord injury the inhibiting outflow is blocked, so the sympathetic innervation continues.

H. Some Syndromes of Incomplete Cord Transection

1. Brown-Séquard Syndrome
—Results from an injury to only half the spinal cord, such as an open penetrating wound producing a hemisection of the cord.
—Characterized by unilateral motor paralysis (corticospinal tract), on the same side as the injury, loss of pain, temperature and touch sensation on the opposite side (spinothalamic tracts), below the site of the injury.
—If it is a lower motor neuron lesion, flaccid muscle tone will be present. If it is an upper motor neuron lesion, spastic muscle tone will prevail.
—Basically, the limb with the best motor functioning will have the least sensation, and the limb with the least motor power will have the best sensation.
—Brown-Séquard syndrome has been reported following heroin injection. It is thought to result from a chemical cord transection due to the heroin or quinine diluent or both, which was injected into an external jugular vein.

2. Anterior Cord Syndrome
—Often associated with cervical flexion trauma, where the anterior section of the cord is injured the most severely.

—Characterized by complete motor paralysis below the level of injury (corticospinal tracts). There is also loss of pain, temperature and touch sensations (spinothalamic tracts). Hyperesthesia and hypalgesia are present. There is some preservation of touch, pressure, position, and vibration.

3. Central Cord Syndrome
—Usually results from a hyperextension injury, where most of the injury is in the central area of the spinal cord.
—The arms have more motor loss than the legs, since the tracts lying centrally in the cord supply the arms. The lumbar and sacral segments lie peripherally in the cord, supplying the legs and bladder. There may also be some sensory impairment in the upper extremities.

V. PSYCHOLOGICAL CONSIDERATIONS

There are certain emotions felt by patients with a spinal cord injury. Various authors give them different names, but essentially they are the following:

Stage I—Shock and Disbelief
This stage has the patient more concerned with whether he will live or die than whether he will walk again. Patient and staff both may be overwhelmed with the medical technology and tasks necessary to get him through the first few days of a catastrophic injury.

Stage II—Denial
This stage is an attempt to escape from the reality of what has happened. The whole realization is too much to handle yet. Sometimes the patient will use partial denial, where he recognizes some of the injury consequences but not others. For instance, the patient may acknowledge that today he can't walk or feel his legs, but given some therapy, he is sure he will be back riding his motorcycle in a couple of months.

The best approach the staff can use during this stage is to focus on the here and now. For instance, focus on today's therapy or learning to do weight shifts instead of on long-term plans for a wheelchair ramp in his home.

Stage III—Reaction
The impact of the injury is fully acknowledged during this phase and the reaction to it is expressed. There may be anger, expressed by verbal or physical abuse, helplessness, often expressed in suicidal statements, depression, and loss of motivation or interest in anything. There may be sexual acting out or alcohol or drug abuse.

Limits may need to be established by the staff to avoid harm to them and to the patient himself. Situations in which the patient might fail should not be introduced at this time. Reinforcement of activities he can do well should be made. Simply listening to the patient express his feelings may be helpful too.

Stage IV—Mobilization
This stage represents the time the patient is actively seeking information about his injury and his self-care. Problem solving between staff, patient and family is seen during this time.

Stage V—Coping
In this stage, the patient learns to live with the neurologic deficits. The resulting disability is no longer the center of the patient's life and thoughts. Interest in other things returns.

VI. GENERAL TREATMENT

A. Medical Management

1. Surgical Intervention
—Spine may need to be stabilized surgically in presence of an unstable injury, especially when the injury is incomplete.
—Surgery is indicated when there is an open injury of the cord, as from a gunshot wound.
—Signs of progressive neurologic deficits may indicate that the means of stabilization is not adequate and surgical intervention should be initiated.
—Surgical management may consist of laminectomy and fusion, insertion of Harrington rods, or anterior fusion.

2. Nonsurgical Intervention
—Spinal alignment may be accomplished with skull tongs (Gardner-Wells, Crutchfield, Vinke, Barton, and Trippi-Wells), in which case the patient is placed on a turning frame.
—A halo brace is another option for cervical spine immobility.
—Intubation and mechanical ventilation may be necessary initially or permanently. Nurses should ensure that the patient has an adequate airway and should monitor respiratory pattern and rate, chest expansion, nasal flaring and use of accessory muscle, breath sounds, ability to clear upper airway with a cough, ventilatory parameters, cyanosis, and arterial blood gases.
—Subtle concomitant head injury should be watched for. Many go undiagnosed in patients with SCI. Head injuries may be most likely to occur concomitantly with traumatic SCI induced by sports accidents, bicycle and motor vehical accidents, and falls. Signs of easy fatigability, memory impairment, trouble with concentration, and irritability may indicate a mild head injury.
—Evaluate specific energy requirements for the patient and supply it through parenteral hyperalimentation if the patient is unable to tolerate oral feedings. Depression and limited mobility can decrease appetite.
—Antispasmotic agents, such as dantrolene sodium (Dantrium) and phenoxybenzamine hydrochloride (Dibenzyline), may be required if the patient is incontinent of urine between catheterizations due to bladder spasms.

—Urological workup is important to determine what type of bladder dysfunction is present. With that information, there should be discussion with the patient regarding his options for long-term bladder management.

—A bowel training regimen should begin on admission to the hospital. The specific program will depend on whether the patient has an automatic reflex bowel (UMN injury) or an autonomous bowel (LMN lesion).

—Hypotension during the spinal shock phase may be treated with vasopressors. Avoid fluid overload.

—Sexual dysfunction based on the level of the lesion should be explained to the patient, and the options for sexual function available. Table 7.1 describes sexual responses possible in patients with different levels of injury.

—Begin range of motion for the patient as soon as possible to break up depositions of bone in connective tissue to prevent or minimize development of heterotopic ossification. Surgical excision of the heterotopic bone may be necessary if range of motion becomes impaired.

—Local cooling of the spinal cord immediately after injury is still experimental, but may hold some hope for minimizing long-term neurologic deficits.

—Hyperbaric oxygen therapy is a treatment in which the patient is put under increased atmospheric pressure and breathes pure oxygen. The purpose is to reverse the progressive ischemic effect of SCI. The results are rather controversial as yet.

—Anticoagulation is a controversial aspect of SCI management. Some studies show less incidence of deep vein thrombosis in heparinized patients, and others demonstrate no significant difference.

—Physical and emotional benefits of sports for helping rehabilitate patients with SCI are well described in the literature. Team sports as well as individual competition may be suggested. Sporting events are also a means to community integration.

—Functional electrical stimulation (FES) of paralyzed muscles is being used in some centers. FES-assisted walking may require less energy from paraplegic patients with complete lesions than the swing-to or swing-through gaits using knee-ankle foot orthoses, since the patients using FES do not have to lift their whole body weight during ambulation. (Fig. 7.1).

—Electrical stimulation is being used in some centers to relieve spasticity in some patients, although the rationale for its use is not well documented.

—If spasticity is severe and interferes with function, surgery or intrathecal injections may be considered.

—Heat/cold applications, vibration, biofeedback, and relaxation techniques are also useful in treating spasticity.

—Pharmacological treatment of spasticity may include the use of benzodiazephines, dantrolene sodium, and baclofen.

Table 7.1.
Sexual Response of Persons with Spinal Cord Injury (Complete Lesion)*

Location of Spinal Cord Injury	General Function	Sexual Function
C1-C3	Severe breathing problems from paralysis of diaphragm and respiratory muscles. Requires artificial ventilation. Usually has neck control and can activate electric wheelchair. No feeling or function below neck.	*Male:* Reflex erection from stimulation of genital region or thighs likely. Psychogenic erection from sexual thoughts not possible. Erogenous areas may develop above line of injury. No change in libidinal drive. *Female:* Little study done. If lubrication analogous to erection, expect reflex lubrication similar to reflexogenic erection. As in male, will not feel sensations or be aware of lubrication unless it is pointed out. No change in libidinal drive. Fertility retained.
C4-C5	Can breathe without artificial ventilation. Needs electric wheelchair and assistance of devices. No feeling or function below clavicle. Can usually dress upper trunk with assistance of devices.	*Male:* Reflex erection likely. Psychogenic erection impossible. Extragenital erogenous zones above level of injury likely. Nongenital orgasm reported. No ejaculation. Oral sex with partner possible. No change in libidinal drive. *Female:* Reflex lubrication likely. Psychogenic lubrication unlike. Extragenital erogenous zones above level of injury likely. Nongenital orgasm reported. Oral sex with partner possible. No change in libidinal drive. Fertility retained.
C6	Most common level of injury.	*Male:* As for C4-C5 level of *(continued)*

*Cord damage may be above or below the level of the bone injury; therefore, two patients with reportedly the same level of injury may have different capabilities. Patients with incomplete lesions may evidence mixtures of abilities. This table provides guidelines, not absolutes. (Reproduced by permission from Weinberg J: Human Sexuality and Spinal Cord Injury. *Nursing Clinics of North America,* Sept. 1982, p 408–409.)

Table 7.1.
(Continued)

Location of Spinal Cord Injury	General Function	Sexual Function
	May use manual chair for short distances. Use of shoulder girdle deltoids and biceps. Loss of deep tendon reflexes and loss of sensation below clavicle.	injury. Holding and caressing now possible. *Female:* As for C4-C5 level of injury. Holding and caressing now possible. Fertility retained.
C7-C8	Can work with hands without assistance of devices. Totally independent in wheelchair transfers.	*Male and female:* Increased potential for use of hands to give pleasure to self and partner.
T1	Called high paraplegia. Full use of hands and fingers. Poor sitting balance.	*Male and female:* As for C7-C8 level of injury but with increased dexterity.
T2-T5	Feeling from level of diaphragm. Upper trunk more mobile.	*Male and female:* Commonly reported orgasmic experiences from nipple stimulation. Reflex erection and lubrication not seen.
T6-T12	May be able to use braces for standing. May participate in strenuous sports. May breathe with chest muscles.	*Male:* Generally still unable to have psychogenic erection. Also unlikely to have reflex erection. *Female:* Water-soluble lubricant needed for intercourse because of decreased reflex lubrication. Libidinal drive remains same. Fertility retained.
L1-L2	May become functionally ambulatory using braces and crutches.	*Male:* Psychogenic stimulation and erection possible between T12 and L2 level of injury. Reflex erections possible but unlikely below L1 and L2. *Female:* Psychogenic erection of clitoris, lubrication, labial swelling, and skin flush possible but unlikely. Fertility retained.

Table 7.1.
(Continued)

Location of Spinal Cord Injury	General Function	Sexual Function
L3-L4	Hip and knee muscles have feeling.	*Male and female:* No reflexogenic erection or lubrication. Psychogenic genital sexual reactions unlikely.
L5-S1	Use of hip, knee, ankle, and foot muscles. No feeling in sexual organs.	*Male and female:* Extragenital sexual potentials great. Erection and lubrication unlikely either through reflexogenic or psychogenic means.
S2-S4	May have bladder and bowel continence.	*Male:* Reflex erection possible. Ejaculation possible (may be retrograde).

—Percutaneous radiofrequency rhizotomy reduces noxious input to the spinal cord, thereby decreasing stimuli that enhance spasticity. It is a relatively new procedure in treatment of spasticity.

—Laser stimulation may be used to reduce spasticity. It is also thought that this new treatment may rechannel brain messages from damaged to healthy nerves. Some patients who had had no somatosensory evoked potentials showed significant positive changes following laser stimulation in some studies.

—A phrenic nerve stimulator may be considered for use in high-level quadriplegics. This is an electronic device that paces the diaphragm via the phrenic nerve. Some advantages of this over a long-term mechanical ventilator are:

• It produces negative pressure ventilation rather than positive pressure, so there is no deleterious effect on circulation.

• A tracheostomy tube may not be necessary or, if present, it may be plugged, so there is less chance for a pulmonary infection and talking is easier. Many physicians recommend that a back-up ventilator be available to the patient and many prefer to have the patient on the ventilator at night. Some research indicates that the phrenic nerve has a limited pacing life and that the diaphragm may fatigue with 24-hour-a-day use.

—Medical management of additonal pathology in a patient with an SCI may be difficult and challenging.

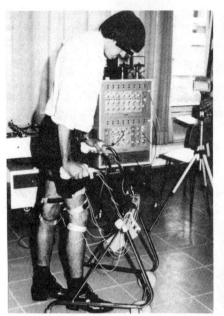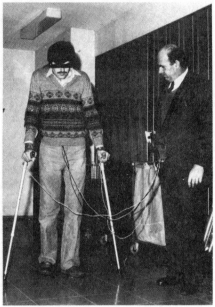

Figure 7.1. Paraplegic patient walking with a four-channel stimulator and walker (left) and with crutches (right). (Reproduced with permission from Bajd T: The Use of a Four-Channel Electrical Stimulator as an Ambulatory Aid for Paraplegic Patients, *Physical Therapy* 63(7): 1119, 1983.)

- The most common complaint of abdominal pathology in patients with SCI is anorexia.
- Pain may or may not be a presenting complaint. If it is present, it is often poorly localized and the patient expresses feelings that "something is wrong." Pain may be referred from the stomach, duodenum or gallbladder to the intrascapular area. Pain from the appendix is often referred to the umbilicus area and kidney pain is referred to the testes or inner thigh.
- Tachycardia may be the only sign of an inflammatory process.
—Spinal-cord-injured patients who have a history of recurrent urinary tract infections or who complain of restlessness, sudden urinary incontinence, and pain in the testes or inner thigh may have pyelonephritis.
- In the absence of recognizable symptoms, patients with SCI may delay seeking medical care.

3. Medical Mangement of Autonomic Dysreflexia
—Elevate the head of the bed.
—Identify and remove the stimulus:
- Empty a distended bladder.

- If impaction is the offending stimulus, apply a local anesthetic agent such as dibucaine ointment (Nupercainal) to the anus and at least one inch into the rectum.
- If pressure sores are the source of the stimulation a position change may relieve it.
- If sexual activity is the stimulus, genital stimulation should be stopped.
- Antispasmotic drugs may be used if an irritated visceral stimulus or bladder spasms are suspected.

—Monitor blood pressure.
—A ganglionic blocking drug such as diazoxide (Hyperstat) may be given intravenously.
—Hydralazine may be administered.

B. Diagnostic Tests

—Spine x-rays are usually done on admission to the hospital.
—Myelography to determine extent of the cord damage, and to identify the site of cord compression.
—Tomography can be useful.
—Serial pulmonary function tests may be indicated in patients with high cervical injuries.
—Neurodiagnostic testing may be used to evaluate cognitive functioning, especially if an occult head injury is suspected in a patient with an SCI.
—The urological workup may include several specific diagnostic tests.

SUGGESTED READINGS

Adelstein W, Watson P. Cervical Spine Injuries. *J Neurosurg Nsg.* 15(2): 65–71, 1983.
Giubilato R. Acute care of the high-level quadriplegic patient. *J Neurosurg Nsg.* 14(3): 128–132, 1982.
Pallett P, O'Brien M. *Textbook of Neurological Nursing.* Boston, Little, Brown, 1985.
Richmond Therese. The patient with a cervical spinal cord injury. *Focus on Crit Care* 12(2): 23–33, April 1985.
Rudy, Ellen. *Advanced Neurological and Neurosurgical Nursing.* St. Louis, CV Mosby, 1984.
Weinberg J. Human sexuality and spinal cord injury. *Nurs Clin America* 17(3): 407–419, 1982.

CHAPTER 8

Central Nervous System Tumors

I. DEFINITION AND DISCUSSION

Tumors within the central nervous system (CNS) often elude early detection during routine health examinations. Tumors may occur in the brain, the spinal cord, or in peripheral nerves. Several body systems may be affected by the presence of a CNS tumor. Numerous neurologic deficits may result, depending upon the location of the pathology.

The health perception-health management functional health pattern is often altered in a patient with this disease process. The potential for injury is present due to frequent loss of coordination, loss of motor skills, sensory-perceptual impairment, cognitive alteration, or other deficits, depending on the tumor location. The treatment of tumors is not without its risks and side effects. Immunosuppressive therapy may in itself place the patient at risk for injury in terms of infection or alteration of the immune system. Malnutrition may also result because of the nausea or anorexia seen after some treatments.

So health management may be difficult to establish or continue in the presence of numerous obstacles. There is certainly a role for nurses in helping patients with CNS tumors, but the long-term outcome may vary.

II. BRAIN TUMORS

A. General Information

—Brain tumors occur in all age groups but more are seen in the 5–8 and 55–60 year age groups.
—There is a slightly higher incidence among males.
—Incidence is higher in whites than in blacks.
—Seventy-five per cent of tumors in adults are supratentorial and of the primary type. Twenty per cent of all primary tumors occur in children. In children, 70% of tumors are infratentorial and most are intraaxial.

—Cerebral tumors account for 1% of all deaths in the United States and 2% of all yearly cancer deaths.

—27,000 new brain tumors are diagnosed each year.

—There are 15,000 deaths each year due to intracranial neoplasms.

—Some tumors occur more commonly in children (cerebellar tumors).

B. Etiology

—Etiology is generally unclear.

—Some factors thought to be related to occurrence of brain tumors are:
- Chemical carcinogens.
- Trauma.
- Radiation.
- Diet.
- Viruses.
- Immunosuppression.
- Genetic factors.

C. Classification

—Classification of brain tumors is done in several different manners. They may be classified by anatomic location, by cellular differentiation (grading), by cellular origin, by whether they are benign or malignant, by whether they are primary or secondary, or according to intraaxial verses extraaxial location.

1. Primary or Secondary Tumors

—Approximately 90% of brain tumors are primary, meaning they developed from CNS tissue. These rarely metastasize outside the CNS.

—Secondary tumors metastasize from other areas of the body, such as the lungs, breast, ovaries, gastrointestinal tract, or kidneys.

2. Intraaxial versus Extraaxial Location (Fig. 8.1)

—Intraaxial tumors are those originating from glial cells. This tissue is within the central neuraxis (cerebrum, cerebellum, brainstem). These tumors affect the brain through infiltration and invasion.

—Extraaxial tumors originate outside the central neuraxis, in the skull, meninges, cranial nerves, and pituitary. The effect on the brain is compression. These tumors can sometimes be more easily excised because they have a superficial location.

3. Cellular Differentiation (Grading)

—Tumors are graded according to the amount of cellular differentiation. The better the cellular differentiation, the better the prognosis.
- Grade I—well-differentiated cells
- Grade II—moderately differentiated cells

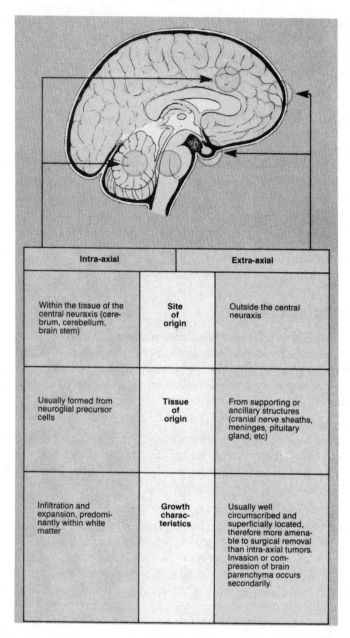

	Intra-axial		Extra-axial
	Within the tissue of the central neuraxis (cerebrum, cerebellum, brain stem)	**Site of origin**	Outside the central neuraxis
	Usually formed from neuroglial precursor cells	**Tissue of origin**	From supporting or ancillary structures (cranial nerve sheaths, meninges, pituitary gland, etc)
	Infiltration and expansion, predominantly within white matter	**Growth characteristics**	Usually well circumscribed and superficially located, therefore more amenable to surgical removal than intra-axial tumors. Invasion or compression of brain parenchyma occurs secondarily.

Figure 8.1. Intraaxial versus extraaxial neoplasms. Reproduced with permission from Day AL: Brain tumors: a clinical guide. *Hospital Medicine* 20(7): 189, 1984.

- Grade III—poorly differentiated cells
- Grade IV—very poorly differentiated cells

—Grade III and IV tumors are typically malignant.

4. Benign versus Malignant Tumors

—Usually the term "benign" indicates a better prognosis. Brain tumors, however, may be benign in terms of histological exam, but due to the location, may be fatal to the patient. Not all benign tumors are in a surgically accessible area. Consequently, there may be no cure for that individual. The tumor may continue to grow or compress vital areas in the brain.

—A "malignant" tumor often indicates a poor prognosis, but not necessarily poorer than a benign tumor in a vital area of the brain.

5. Cellular Origin

—Tumors may be classified by the specific cell type from which they originate. For example astrocytomas arise from astrocyte cells.

6. Location

  a. *Major Groups of Neoplasms*

   1. Gliomas

- Originate from neuroglial cells.
- Rapidly growing and infiltrative.
- Account for almost half of all intracranial tumors.
- Subclassified into five tumor types, according to predominant glial cell type:

   a) Astrocytoma

   —Account for 38% of all gliomas.

   —Six to 10% are benign (Grade I) but they often undergo cellular change and advance to the malignant glioblastomas (Grade III and IV astrocytoma).

   —May infiltrate large areas of the brain.

   —Signs and symptoms depend on size and location.

   —Grades I and II are slow growing. Grades III and IV are rapid growing.

   —Complete surgical excision rarely possible.

   b) Glioblastoma Multiforme

   —Highly vascular.

   —Most malignant tumor which often invades the temporal and frontal lobes, basal ganglia, and commissural pathways. Rare in the brainstem and cerebellum.

   —Rapid growth causes invasion of adjacent brain tissue and cerebral edema.

   —Average survival in treated patients is 12 to 18 months from onset of clinical symptoms.

   —Occurs in patients 45–55 years of age most often.

   —Represent one-third of all gliomas.

—Comprised of various cell types ("multiforme").

—Signs and symptoms depend on size and location.

—Surgery, chemotherapy to retard growth and radiation therapy do not usually increase survival rate. Surgical resection and decompression may decrease signs of brain compression.

c) Medulloblastoma

—Accounts for 11% of all gliomas.

—Occurs primarily in children, particularly among boys between 6 and 10 years of age.

—Highly malignant and rapidly growing.

—Often invades the fourth ventricle and metastasizes to the subarachnoid spaces of the hemisphere and spinal cord. It produces obstructive hydrocephalus, so signs of increased intracranial pressure may be seen.

—Cerebellar signs and flu-like symptoms are common. Squinting in children may be a sign of visual disturbance.

—Average survival is approximately one year after onset of symptoms.

—Very radiosensitive but whole brain and spinal cord must be radiated because of possibility of malignant cells seeding via the CSF.

d) Ependymoma

—Occurs in children and adolescents primarily.

—Originates from cells within the ventricular system, most often in the fourth ventricle.

—Causes ventricular obstruction and hydrocephalus, so signs of increased ICP may be seen (see Chapter 2).

—Survival is about 3 years.

—Represents about 6% of all gliomas.

—Most are benign but may become malignant.

—Grades I and II respond poorly to radiation but Grades III and IV may benefit.

e) Oligodendroglioma

—Makes up fewer than 5% of all gliomas.

—Often located in the hemispheres of young adults or the thalamus of children.

—May be slow growing and produce long-term focal problems or may present rapidly with associated hemorrhage. The patient often has a long history of seizures (first symptom in 50% of patients).

—Skull x-rays may demonstrate a densely calcified, well-defined mass. The tumor may be diffusely infiltrated, however. Recurrence is frequent.

—Survival in some studies is 10–15 years with surgery and radiation. Other studies report a 21 month survival.

—Radical surgery is often followed by radiation.

3. Metastatic Tumors

—Represent 20% of all brain tumors.

—Occur most often in middle-aged or older adults with a previously diagnosed primary cancer outside the CNS.

—Most often come from lesions of the bronchus (especially with the current increased incidence of lung cancer) or the breast. May also result from a primary site in the gastrointestinal tract, kidney, ovary, or from a melanoma.

—Supratentorial metastases result in seizures, focal signs, and signs of increased ICP. Infratentorial metastases result in cerebellar signs (ataxia, vertigo, vomiting, and headache from the hydrocephalus). Infiltration of the cauda equina may cause paresthesia of the legs and bowel and bladder dysfunction.

—The metastases usually spread via the arterial system and lodge at the junction of the gray and white matter, where rapid expansion occurs beneath the cortical surface. This results in profound white matter edema with a mass effect. The patient may die from the increased ICP and not from the primary tumor.

—Surgery is a palliative treatment.

b. *Less Frequently Occurring Brain Tumors*

1. Acoustic Neuroma (Schwannoma or Neurofibroma)

—Originates from the sheath of Schwann cells in the vestibular portion of the eighth cranial nerve.

—Benign.

—Encapsulated.

—Accounts for 5% of intracranial tumors.

—Slow growing.

—Usually located at the cerebellopontine angle, causing unilateral cranial nerve symptoms.

—Other symptoms may include ataxia, signs of increased ICP from hydrocephalus, deafness, rotational vertigo, facial numbness, weakness, paralysis, tinnitus, loss of extraocular eye movements, drooling, drooping of one side of the mouth, difficulty swallowing, loss of corneal reflex.

—May compress fifth and seventh cranial nerves. Large tumors may involve ninth and tenth cranial nerves and cerebellum.

—Complete removal of small tumors results in excellent prognosis. With incomplete excision there is a 30% mortality in 3–4 years. Fifty percent of patients with incomplete removal have recurrence.

2. Pituitary Adenomas

—Represent 7–10% of primary intracranial neoplasms.

—Encapsulated.

—Present most often between ages of 30–40 years.

—Benign.

—Subdivided into three types according to cell type:

a) Chromophobic Pituitary Adenoma

   —Most common of the three types of pituitary adenomas (90% of all pituitary tumors).

   —Usually contained within the posterior fossa.

   —Nonsecreting tumor.

   —Causes hypopituitarism by compressing and injuring the anterior region of the pituitary gland.

   —Results in amenorrhea, loss of libido, sterility in females, and impotence in males due to decreased gonadotropin secretion.

   —Other symptoms include visual impairment and bitemporal hemianopia from optic chiasm compression.

   —Microadenomas of the anterior pituitary may cause excessive prolactin secretion, which would result in galactorrhea and irregularities of the menstrual cycle in females and oligospermia and impotence in males.

   —Diabetes insipidus occurs in 5% of patients.

   —Surgical removal beneficial using transphenoidal microsurgery for pituitary tumors.

b) Basophilic Pituitary Adenoma

   —Secretes an excess of corticotropin, which causes Cushing's syndrome (moon faces, "buffalo hump," truncal obesity, hypertension, abdominal stria, diabetes mellitus, thin arms and legs, osteoporosis, muscle weakness, amenorrhea or impotence, pendulous abdomen, elevated ACTH levels).

   —Ergot derivatives such as bromocriptine control some hypersecreting pituitary states.

c) Eosinophilic (Acidophilic) Pituitary Adenoma

   —Secretes excessive amounts of growth hormone. Produces gigantism if it occurs before the bone epiphyses have fused (after puberty). In an adult it results in acromegaly (enlarged hands and feet, prominent forehead and lower jaw, thickening of soft tissue, especially of facial features, separation of teeth, visual loss, diabetes mellitus, course hair and skin, hyperphosphatemia, large tongue, hypercalciuria, joint pain, hypertension, hyperhidrosis, and visceral organ enlargement, such as the heart).

   —Surgical debulking and radiation may be combined for treatment of large tumors.

3. Craniopharyngiomas

   —Make up approximately 3% of all intracranial tumors.

—Occur most frequently in children and in males.

—Solid or cystic tumors.

—Congenital. Symptoms occur before age 15 in 50% of cases.

—Benign.

—Originate from remnants of the hypophyseal duct. They are located above the sella turcica and depress the optic chiasm and often extend into the third ventricle; may obstruct flow of CSF.

—Symptoms include those of increased ICP due to hydrocephalus, visual disturbances, vertigo, seizures, hemiparesis, mental deterioration, pituitary hypofunction, and diabetes insipidus. In children, there may be impairment of body growth and maturation.

—Almost all tumors recur after surgical intervention. It may be due to their insinuation into so many structures that some cells are left behind.

—Resection may be by transphenoidal or intracranial approach.

—Radiation sensitive after surgery.

4. Hemangioblastomas

—Slow growing.

—Vascular.

—Occur most often in the cerebellum.

—Most frequently present in patients during ages 40–50.

—Tend to run in families.

—Symptoms include cerebellar signs and polycythemia (because they secrete erythropoietin).

—Surgery may be useful with radiation therapy if there is recurrence.

5. Cholesteatomas

—Slow growing epidermoid tumors.

—Usually detected in young adults.

—Benign, but may spread throughout the brain making complete excision impossible.

6. Pseudotumor Cerebri (Benign Intracranial Hypertension)

—Characterized by increased intracranial pressure, usually in the absence of neurologic manifestations other than headache, papilledema, and sometimes visual disturbances.

—This syndrome may follow an ear infection, an endocrine disorder, hormone or drug therapy, hypervitaminosis A, or withdrawal of steroid therapy.

—Frequently occurs in young obese females who have a history of irregular menstrual cycles.

7. Chordomas

—Malignant.

—Slow growing.

—Locally invasive.

—Occur usually in males.

—Originate at base of the cranium usually, but can form anywhere in the vertebral column.

—They may destroy bone, invade the dura, and infiltrate the floor of the posterior fossa, resulting in cranial nerve palsies.

—May extend into the ear, neck paranasal sinuses, and nasopharynx.

—Complete surgical removal may be impossible. Chemotherapy may be tried also.

8. Teratomas

—Usually found in children.

—Congenital.

—Infiltrating and difficult to treat.

—Contain residual embryonic tissues such as cartilage, muscle, and intestinal and respiratory epithelium.

—Most common site is in or near the pineal body, near the pituitary, or near the third ventricle.

—They impair endocrine function and may result in early puberty.

—They may impair CSF flow and cause hydrocephalus, resulting in signs of increased ICP.

—Surgery is attempted for space-occupying lesions but may not be successful for infiltrating tumors such as this.

D. Medical Management

1. Surgery

—Tissue biopsy will identify the tumor histologically and provide information toward a prognosis. A biopsy may guide the medical management.

—Some tumors, although histologically benign, are not accessible to surgical intervention. Only partial removal is safe with large infiltrating or very vascular tumors such as glioblastoma multiforme and hemangioblastomas. Partial removal may be performed to decompress the brain and relieve ICP.

—A shunting procedure may be indicated to decompress the ventricular system and relieve intracranial pressure.

—Complete surgical excision is the preferred treatment when possible. This is usually possible if the tumor is small, well-circumscribed, and in an accessible region. Examples of tumors that often meet these criteria are meningiomas, pituitary tumors, acoustic neuromas, and cystic astrocytomas of the cerebellum and third ventricle.

2. Radiation Therapy

—Radiation may be used in addition to surgical intervention and for palliation in metastatic tumors.

—Its purpose is to destroy tumor cells while minimizing the side effects and the effects on normal brain cells.

—Sometimes used in combination with chemotherapy.

3. Chemotherapy

—Most chemotherapeutic agents work by interfering at some stage of cell reproduction, thereby destroying the tumor cell. These agents are not specific, however, for tumor cells, and may affect bone marrow, hair follicles, and the intestinal epithelium. This results in fatigue, hair loss, nausea and vomiting, diarrhea, and increased risk for infection and bleeding.

—Several nitrosourea agents are able to cross the blood-brain barrier and are effective against brain tumors (BCNU, CCNU, and methyl CCNU).

—Intrathecal and intraventricular antineoplastics may be used, such as methotrexate. It is instilled directly into a lateral ventricle through a surgically-implanted reservoir, either with a catheter into the ventricle or into the CSF via a lumbar puncture. Methotrexate has also been given in an intraarterial infusion. Intrathecal administration may cause a headache and fever and sometimes acute encephalopathy. Other side effects include bone marrow depression, nausea and vomiting, mucositis, and diarrhea.

4. Immunotherapy

—The basis for immunotherapy is that a tumor produces an antigen which in a normal host would stimulate production of an antibody, to ward off the foreign antigen. Patients with intracranial tumors have a depressed immune system and this normal action does not take place. Immunotherapy consists of giving a patient drugs by vaccination to enhance the body's immune system or help develop an active immunity to the tumor cells. This has not yet been very successful.

5. Hyperbaric Oxygen Therapy

—Hyperbaric oxygen therapy is based on the premise that hypoxic cells are less sensitive to x-ray injury than are cells in a normal oxygen environment. Many tumor cells have a poor oxygen content. The hyperbaric chamber increases the oxygen tension in the tumor cells so the effects of radiation are enhanced. The results of this therapy are still inconclusive.

6. Drug Therapy

—Steroids are thought to slow tumor growth and reduce cerebral swelling. Dexamthasone (Decadron) is the usual drug of choice. It also helps control radiation edema.

—Cimetadine (Tagamet) is usually given while steroids are being administered to reduce gastric secretions.

—Phenytoin (Dilantin) is often given prophylactically to prevent seizures. The tumor may be a focus for abnormal electrical discharges.

—Some analgesic for headache is given, such as acetaminophen or codeine.

—Stool softeners may be indicated to prevent straining.

—Increased intracranial pressure may be treated with osmotic agents and hyperventilation (see Chapter 2).

E. Diagnostic Tests

—Skull films may demonstrate a deviation of a calcified pineal body by a brain mass, erosion of bone, and calcified areas within a tumor.

—CAT scan gives more information about size and location of a tumor and demonstrates hydrocephalus.

—Visual field and funduscopic exam will reveal visual field cuts and papilledema.

—Angiography will outline the vascularity in the brain and in the tumor.

—Electroencephalogram (EEG) may help localize a lesion. Seventy-five percent of patients with brain tumors have abnormal EEG tracings.

—A brain scan will help define a mass. Brain tumors impair the blood-brain barrier so there is increased uptake of radioactive isotope within the tumor.

—If a lumbar puncture is deemed necessary, the CSF protein will usually be elevated in one-third of patients with intracranial neoplasms. Cytological exam may show cancerous cells.

—Biopsy will give a more definitive diagnosis of tumor type.

—Audiometric tests and abnormal caloric test (occluvestibular reflex) suggest acoustic neuroma. Cisternal myelogram with tomography may be needed to visualize the cerebellopontine angle.

—Pituitary tumors are detected with endocrinologic, ophthalmologic, and radiologic studies. Radioimmunoassays determine the amount of circulating pituitary hormones. Insulin tolerance testing and 24-hour urine tests for steroids are also available. Coned x-ray views and polytomograms of the sella turcica are done to detect erosion, ballooning, or other irregularities. Prolactin levels are drawn to help diagnose a prolactin-secreting tumor.

—Chest x-rays and other routine studies may be done to try to find the primary tumor site.

—A cisternogram will reveal presence of hydrocephalus when tumors tend to obstruct the circulation of CSF.

—Endocrine tests may be especially abnormal with pituitary adenomas and craniopharyngiomas.

—Positron emission tomography (PET scan) illustrates the metabolism of the tumor and surrounding brain tissue.

—Tumor markers are substances made by the tumor cells which are sometimes very specific or unique to a particular class of tumor. By measuring these markers in blood or cerebrospinal fluid, it is possible to diagnose the tumor type and determine the response to therapy.

III. SPINAL CORD TUMORS

A. General Information

—Ten to 20% of all CNS tumors are located in the spinal cord.

—Fifty per cent of spinal tumors are found in the thoracic region.

—Spinal cord compression caused by a mass lesion usually evolves slowly, in contrast to sudden compression from acute spinal trauma.

—The spinal cord can be damaged both by mechanical pressure placed on it by a mass, or by ischemia that results when arterial blood supply to the cord is compromised by the mass.

—Unlike brain tumors, 85% of intraspinal neoplasms tend to be benign.

—Spinal cord tumors occur equally in both sexes, usually in the 20 to 60 year age range, and they are rarely found before the age of 10 or in the elderly.

B. Classification of Spinal Tumors

—Classification is based on the relationship of the tumor to the dura and the spinal cord, as well as on histological type. (Fig. 8.2)

1. Extradural Tumors

—Originate in the meninges, blood vessels, or in nerve roots and continue outside the cord.

—Most common types are from metastatic growths in the lungs, breast, kidney, prostate, lymphoid tissue, gastrointestinal tract, uterus, and thyroid.

—Chondromas (cartilaginous slow-growing tumors), meningiomas, and neurofibromas (tumors of connective tissue of a nerve), and osteomas are more rare.

—Approximately 90% are malignant, with 75–80% of metastatic origin.

—Rapid onset of symptoms.

—Earliest symptom is usually severe localized back pain or radicular pain. Within weeks or months signs of cord compression become evident (lower extremity numbness or weakness and eventually paraplegia). Most damage is done by compression, although occasionally the tumor may infiltrate the extradural space.

—Vibratory sense and position sense below the tumor level become impaired. Bladder and bowel control is lost later.

—The localized pain is made worse in the recumbent position. This is caused by traction on the diseased nerve root as the spine elongates when the shortening effects of gravity and weight are removed.

—Radicular pain to the dermatomes is made worse by movement, coughing or straining.

—Most extradural tumors are fast growing.

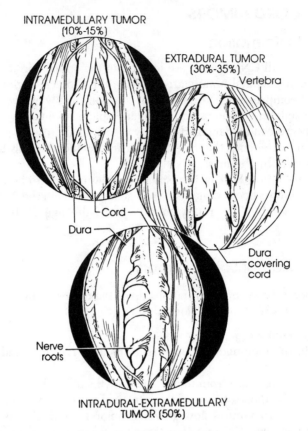

Figure 8.2. Location and frequency of spinal cord tumors—extradural 30% to 35%; intradural 50%; intramedullary 10% to 15%. (Reproduced with permission from Snyder M., Jackle M.: *Neurologic Problems: A Critical Care Nursing Focus,* Bowle, Md., R.J. Brady Co., 1981, p. 346.)

2. **Intradural Spinal Tumors**
    a) *Extramedullary (within the dura but outside the cord itself)*
       —Most commonly occurring spinal tumor.
       —Meningiomas and neurofibromas are the most common types.
       —Occur primarily in fourth and fifth decades.
       —No sex predilection.
       —Occur most frequently in thoracic area.
       —Slow gradual onset.
       —Commonly manifest nerve root symptoms early, and long tract signs later. Local and radicular pain may be present, but not always.
       —Cord compression may be incomplete (e.g., Brown-Séquard's syndrome).

—Meningiomas are often loosely adhering to the dura, making surgical excision easy.

—Neurofibromas originate in the dorsal nerve roots. If they extend on both sides of the intervertebral foramen, they may take on the classic "dumb-bell" or "hour-glass" shape. Sometimes these tumors are part of a generalized neurofibromatosis.

b) *Intramedullary*

—Located within the spinal cord itself.

—Almost 95% are gliomas arising from neuroglia rather than from nerve tissue itself.

—Most common types are the ependymomas (originating mainly in the lumbar and cauda equina areas) and astrocytomas (originating mainly in the cervical area).

—Ependymomas are twice as frequent as astrocytomas.

—Slow growing with progressive onset of symptoms.

—Paralysis, sensory loss and bladder dysfunction are frequent. If the tumor is in the caudal area, there will be bowel, bladder, and sexual dysfunction. Areflexia, muscle weakness and atrophy may be demonstrated. Pain may be severe if the tumor compresses spinal roots or vertebrae, but usually the compression is on the center fiber tracts of the cord. There may be bilateral segmental loss of pain and temperature sensation.

C. Medical Management

—Surgical excision is the usual treatment choice, often in combination with radiation and/or chemotherapy. Surgery is done to relieve spinal cord or nerve root compression. It is a palliative measure with malignant and non-removable tumors.

—Analgesics are necessary for pain control.

—If radiation is used, radiation myelopathy is a potential complication that should be observed for. There is an insidious onset of sensory impairment to areas innervated by the affected cord. Motor symptoms and changes in pain and temperature occur, so a Brown-Séquard syndrome may be seen. A spastic paraplegia, loss of sensation and loss of bowel and bladder function usually result. This occurs about 6 months after completion of the therapy.

—Cord edema may be controlled with dexamethasone (Decadron). Cimetadine (Tagamet) is given during steroid administration.

—Rehabilitation may be aggressive or moderate, depending on the patient's needs.

—Cordotomy or palliative section of the sensory roots may be done for intractable pain.

—A shunting procedure may be done for hydrocephalus, which may develop as a result of impaired CSF resorption pathways due to the elevated CSF protein level present with most spinal tumors.

D. Diagnostic Tests

—Spinal x-rays and tomograms are done.
—Myelography helps localize the tumor. Cord compression can be seen when contrast medium is introduced into the spinal canal.
—If a lumbar puncture is done, there is an elevated level of protein in the CSF. There is a risk of causing increased cord compression due to changing the CSF pressure below the tumor.
—CAT scanning with a contrast medium also helps visualize the cord compression.
—Since the spinal tumor may be secondary, a workup to find the primary site is performed (chest x-rays, breast exam, blood work etc.)
—The Quechenstedt test is positive if the tumor is encroaching upon the subarachnoid space. This test demonstrates a spinal subarachnoid obstruction with compression of the jugular veins bilaterally.
—If a vascular tumor is suspected, spinal angiography may be done.
—Electromyography (EMG) may help rule out multiple sclerosis and amyotrophic lateral sclerosis.
—Two conditions that mimic spinal tumors are:
  • Spinal abscesses
    —Somewhat rare.
    —Usually caused by a bacteremia.
    —Symptoms occur suddenly with localized pain and tenderness over the involved spinal area.
    —Treatment involves surgical drainage and antibiotics.
  • Syringomyelia
    —In this condition there is cavitation and scar tissue which forms within the central cord canal.
    —Cavitation causes injury to pain and temperature fibers and also impairs some autonomic responses.
    —Considered a congenital problem, although clinical signs do not appear until about age 30.
    —Air myelography will reveal a "collapsing cord" which is typical of this disorder. The cord with an intramedullary tumor does not change shape regardless of the position the patient assumes.
    —No specific treatment for this degenerative disease.

SUGGESTED READINGS

American Association of Neuroscience Nursing Core Curriculum, Park Ridge, Il., Am. Assoc. of Neuroscience Nursing, 1984.

Arsenault L: Primary spinal cord tumors: a review and case presentation of a patient with an intramedullary spinal cord neoplasm. *J Neurosurg* 13(2): 53–58, 1981.

Day A: Brain tumors: a clinical guide. *Hospital Med* 20(7): 188–216, 1984.

Hickey J: *The Clinical Practice of Neurological and Neurosurgical Nursing.* Philadelphia, JB Lippincott, 1981.

Pallett P, O'Brien M: *Textbook of Neurological Nursing.* Boston, Little, Brown, 1985.

Rudy E.: *Advanced Neurological and Neurosurgical Nursing.* St. Louis, Mosby, 1984.

CHAPTER 9

Neurologic Infectious Disorders

I. DEFINITION AND DISCUSSION

A central nervous system infectious disorder may be a complication of another injury, such as meningitis being a complication of a traumatic head injury, or it may be a separate process. Infection may be from many different organisms: bacteria, parasites, or viruses being the most common. A central nervous system infection often causes edema within the cranial cavity or spinal cord. This edema may cause secondary injury to neurons. So neuronal injury or infarction is certainly a possible result of an infectious process.

Patients with neurologic disorders or injuries may be at risk for infection for several reasons. Some may be immunosuppressed. Many receive steroids, and some receive chemotherapy or radiation therapy. Some have had multiple trauma injuries and have had surgical intervention for various reasons. There is always the possibility of a nosocomial infection once the patient is hospitalized. Patients may become nutritionally depleted if care is not taken to continually assess caloric need and caloric intake. When a patient's gastrointestinal tract is not able to be used for nutrition, it is vital that calories are provided in another manner, such as total parenteral nutrition. If nutrition is neglected, healing slows and the patient's ability to fight infection is diminished.

II. ETIOLOGY AND PATHOPHYSIOLOGY

A. General Information

1. **Meningitis**
—May be due to bacteria, virus, yeast, or fungus.
—Most common organisms causing meningitis are *Hemophilus influenzae,* *Neisseria meningitidis,* and *Streptococcus pneumoniae.* These organisms cause 80–90% of all cases of bacterial meningitis.
—Meningitis is an inflammatory reaction within the pia and arachnoid

meninges. The infection is carried via the cerebrospinal fluid (CSF) to the entire brain and spinal cord.

—The infection is most often introduced to the central nervous system from the bloodstream or from contiguous infected areas such as the sinuses or middle ear, or from penetrating head injuries and skull fractures.

—Nosocomial meningitis is rare but may result from contamination of the CSF during a lumbar puncture or neurosurgical operative procedures.

—Meningitis occurs worldwide. Incidence is fairly constant, except for a small decrease in incidence during summer months.

—*Hemophilus influenzae* meningitis is most common in the 3-month to 7-year age range. Children and teenagers have a higher incidence of meningococcal meningitis. Pneumococcal meningitis is most frequent in the very young and those over 40 years old.

—Signs and symptoms include:
  • Headache—usually the first symptom. This is a result of irritation to the pain-sensitive dura and traction on cerebral vasculature.
  • Fever—may be masked initially if the patient is receiving steroids.
  • Meningeal signs—nuchal rigidity, positive Brudzinski's sign and positive Kernig's sign.
  • Changes in level of consciousness—may become delerious, restless, combative, lethargic, incoherent, or unresponsive.
  • Photophobia.
  • Seizures—due to cortical irritation. May also be a result of high doses of antibiotics if the patient is already being treated.
  • Increased intracranial pressure may result from a developing hydrocephalus or cerebral swelling.
  • Irritability.
  • Nausea and vomiting.

—Viral or aseptic meningitis may not cause severe changes in level of consciousness. Resolution is in 10–14 days, usually with no sequelae in over 90% of cases. Mumps virus is the usual causative organism.

—Tuberculous meningitis occurs mostly in young children in areas of the world where tuberculosis is prevalent. In areas of the world where tuberculosis is not prevalent, tuberculous meningitis usually affects the elderly who develop a reactivation of a dormant infection.

—Fungal meningitis usually occurs in immunologically deficient patients.

2. Encephalitis

—Encephalitis is an inflammation of the brain parenchyma.

—May be caused by a virus, bacteria, rickettsia, fungus, or a parasite.

—Acute viral encephalitis is often caused by arbovirus and herpes simplex infections.

  a. *Arbovirus encephalitis*
    • Transmitted by mosquitoes or ticks.

- Residual effects may include mental retardation, dementia, paresis or paralysis, deafness, blindness, epilepsy, and personality changes with psychosis.

b. *Herpes simplex encephalitis*
   - Most common form of encephalitis.
   - High fatality rate.
   - Diagnosis may be difficult because symptoms are similar to acute functional psychosis, meningitis, subarachnoid hemorrhage, tumor, or abscess.
   - Usually causes extensive neuronal damage of the hemispheres, mostly gray matter.
   - Clinical features include fever, headache, seizures, hemiparesis, nuchal rigidity, ataxia, dysphasia, altered mental status, difficulty chewing or swallowing, blurred vision, diplopia, and facial muscle weakness.
   - Frontal and temporal lobes are most frequently involved sites.
   - A serious complication of herpes simplex encephalitis can be a residual syndrome in which the patient demonstrates fluent dysphasia and inability to incorporate new information.

c. *Postviral diseases which may result in a central nervous system infection include measles, mumps, and chickenpox.*

3. Cysticerosis
—The most common parasite affecting the central nervous system.
—Systemic infection caused by the encysted larval form of tapeworm.
—Changing immigration patterns are causing an increased frequency of this disorder in the United States.
—Five years is the average time between initial infection and onset of symptoms.
—Humans are infected by eating undercooked or raw pork, which may contain tapeworms. The tapeworm grows in the human gastrointestinal tract, penetrates the alimentary canal and enters the blood stream. The brain, eye and/or skeletal muscles are invaded. Once lodged in an organ, the organism forms a cyst, 3–15 mm in diameter. The cyst holds larva. The larva eventually die (about 18 months after infection), and the cyst becomes calcified. An inflammatory reaction results.
—Obstructive hydrocephalus and arterial thrombosis are severe complications. Embolization into the cerebral vasculature can obstruct blood flow and cause cerebral infarction.
—Multiple cysts may be present in a person's brain and they may appear radiologically to be one mass.

4. Reye's Syndrome
—Worldwide distribution, affecting both sexes.
—Mortality rates differ, but nationally, is about 40–50%.

—Affects Caucasian children from rural or suburban areas more often than other ethnic groups. Black children under one year of age from lower socio-economic urban areas reportedly are affected more than white infants.

—Affects children mostly between birth and age of 19 years, with peaks at ages 6 and 11.

—Late winter and early spring are peak seasons for Reye's Syndrome.

—Characterized by an antecedent viral infection that is followed by hepatic, metabolic, and neurologic dysfunctions. Influenza B and varicella are the most common antecedent viral infections.

—Use of aspirin and phenothiazines during the prodromal illness is thought to have a relationship to the occurrence of the syndrome.

—Clinical features may include fever, vomiting, cough, changes in mental status, restlessness, combativeness, visual hallucinations, sympathetic activity (tachycardia, tachypnea, pupil dilatation, sweating), an enlarged liver, seizures, and signs of increased intracranial pressure.

—Prognostic indicators associated with poor outcome from the disease are:
  • Deep stage of coma on admission to a health care facility.
  • Ammonia level over 300 µg/ml.
  • Sustained hyperosmolality over 350 mOsm/L.
  • Sustained hypothrombinemia (less than 30% of control).
  • Severe hypocapnia (PCO_2 below 10 mm Hg).
  • Sustained increased intracranial pressure with a low cerebral perfusion pressure (under 50 mm Hg).

—Theories of etiology include the following:
  • Viral—most victims have a prodromal viral illness, although no virus has yet been isolated.
  • Genetic—some siblings develop the disease, so there may be a genetic predisposition.
  • Toxins—interaction between a virus and a toxin may be the cause of Reye's syndrome. Toxins under close investigation include insecticides and pesticides, metabolites of salicylates, phenothiazines, and decongestants.

—Pathologically there is fatty degeneration of the viscera, especially the liver, but also the kidneys, heart, lungs, skeletal muscle, and pancreas. The primary abnormality lies in the mitochondria.

5. Acquired Immune Deficiency Syndrome (AIDS)

—At least 40% of AIDS victims are neurologically symptomatic. They may develop an opportunistic infection which affects the central nervous system and causes encephalitis, meningitis, and/or seizures. These patients may also develop an encephalopathy secondary to a metabolic disturbance or an opportunistic infection.

—The most current data from the U.S. Department of Health and Human Services and the Public Health Service, in a March 1987 report indicates that 97% of AIDS patients in the United States can be placed in groups related to possible means of disease acquisition: men with homosexual or bisexual orientation who have histories of using intravenous drugs (8% of cases); homosexual or bisexual men who are not known intravenous drug users (65%); heterosexual intravenous drug users (17%); persons with hemophilia (1%); heterosexual sex partners of persons with AIDS or at risk for AIDS (4%); and recipients of transfused blood or blood components (2%). Not enough data are available to classify the remaining 3% by the above recognized risk factors for AIDS.

In Africa over 90% of cases have occurred through heterosexual transmission, equally divided among women and men.

—The AIDS virus has been shown to be spread from an infected person to an unifected person by:
- Sexual contact.
- Sharing of needles used to inject drugs.
- An infected woman to her fetus or newly born baby.
- Transfusion or injection of infectious blood or blood products.

—Clinical features vary. Weight loss, fever, diarrhea, malaise and lymphadenopathy may be demonstrated. Kaposi's sarcoma or other malignant neoplasms may be seen. *Pneumocystis carinni* pneumonia is the usual opportunistic infection (a protozoa-infection). Progressive dementia is a neurologic manifestation often seen. Forgetfulness, personality changes, hemiparesis, seizures, and blindness may occur.

6. Brain Abscess

—Three common areas for suppurative lesions to form are the cerebrum, the subdural space, and the epidural (extradural) space.

—Forty per cent of brain abscesses are caused by middle-ear and mastoid infections. Ten per cent are a result of sinus infections. About 50% are metastatic abscesses, that is, carried by the blood from an infectious site such as from lung infections or abscesses, skin infections or acute bacterial endocarditis.

—Acute clinical manifestations of brain abscess may include headache, malaise, chills and fever, some focal neurologic sign such as lethargy, motor or sensory impairment, speech disorders or seizure activity.

—Clinical manifestations during the stage of enlargement are those caused by a mass lesion: headache, signs of increased intracranial pressure, localized deficits, stupor.

III. GENERAL TREATMENTS: MEDICAL MANAGEMENT AND DIAGNOSTIC TESTS

A. Meningitis

—A lumbar puncture for CSF analysis is helpful in diagnosing meningitis. The CSF opening pressure may be elevated, the protein elevated, the glucose decreased, the color cloudy or xanthochromic.

—The history should include inquiring about recent infection in the ears, sinus or respiratory tract.

—A CAT scan may help identify hydrocephalus, middle-ear or sinus pus collections, or abscesses.

—Skull films may identify a skull fracture or sinus or mastoid diseases.

—Treatment includes use of supportive measures, such as controlling headache, fever, maintaining fluid and electrolyte balance, and preventing seizure activity.

—Antibiotics are given for the specific bacterial organism identified. When an antibiotic is used, it must be able to cross the blood-brain barrier to be effective in this central nervous system infection. Penicillin and its derivatives and chloromycetin have good penetration. Viral meningitis is not treated with antibiotics.

—Meningococcal meningitis is the only one for which isolation is necessary. It is passed by droplet method, so it requires a respiratory isolation until the cultures are negative (usually within 24 hours after antimicrobial therapy is initiated).

B. Encephalitis

—A lumbar puncture is done to analyze the CSF. There may be an elevated opening pressure, xanthochromia from the hemorrhagic nature of the brain lesions, an elevated protein level and white cell count, primarily lymphocytes. The Herpes simplex virus is inactivated at room temperature, so it is difficult to culture the virus from the CSF.

—An EEG may show focal or generalized slowing with some seizure activity or paroxysmal burst activity.

—Brain biopsy may be performed.

—Antibody titers may be useful.

—Herpes encephalitis is treated with adenine arabinoside (Ara-A) intravenously.

—Management of cerebral edema is necessary (see Chapter 2).

—Supportive measures to control pain and temperature are used.

—Steroids may be used except in the case of Herpes simplex encephalitis. Steroids in that disease are thought to increase the spread of herpesvirus through nervous tissue.

C. Cysticercosis

—CAT scan is done to identify cysts.

—A lumbar puncture may be performed so CSF analysis may be done.

—There is a test for serum-indirect hemagglutination titers for cysticercosis. However it reportedly gives about 13% false-positive and 12.5% false-negative results.

—Surgical biopsy may be needed.

—Surgical excision may be performed if the cyst is accessible.

—A shunt may be performed to relieve the obstructive hydrocephalus when the cyst cannot be surgically removed.

—Anticonvulsants are used to prevent seizure activity.

—Steroids may be given to reduce inflammation.

—Praziquantel (Biltricide) is effective in ridding the gastrointestinal tract of tapeworms. In the laboratory it has been shown that this drug can penetrate the wall of the cyst and kill the larva. An inflammatory response may result from use of the drug, probably due to changes induced in the parasite, so that is a therapeutic risk. It must be carefully monitored if the patient has increased intracranial pressure.

—Metrifonate and radioactive antibodies are also available therapies.

D. Reye's Syndrome

—Laboratory results that are consistent with Reye's syndrome are:
  • Hyperammonemia.
  • Elevated serum glutamic oxaloacetic transaminase (SGOT) and serum glutamic pyruvic transaminase (SGPT).
  • Hypoprothrombinemia.
  • Hypoglycemia.
  • Elevated serum amino acid and free fatty acids.
  • Respiratory alkalosis with a metabolic acidosis (due to dehydration from vomiting, hyperventilation, and salicylate intake).
  • Elevated BUN and creatinine.

—EEG may be done. Different readings may be seen during different stages of the disease.

—The clinical history and physical exam are also necessary for diagnosis.

—Treatment involves supportive care to normalize organ function and protect the brain from irreversible injury.
  • Treat increased intracranial pressure (see Chapter 2).
  • Correct fluid and electrolyte abnormalities, acidosis, hypoglycemia, and hypoxia.
  • Barbiturate coma may be instituted (see chapter on intracranial pressure).
  • Treat bleeding with fresh frozen plasma and work up patient for DIC (disseminated intravascular coagulopathy). Vitamin K may be given intravenously.
  • Neomycin may be used to inhibit absorption of ammonia.

E. Acquired Immune Deficiency Syndrome (AIDS)

—There is currently no predictable diagnostic indicator for the disease. The enzyme-linked immunosorbent assay (ELISA) test for detection of antibody production of HIV does, however, identify persons with previous exposure to the virus. The test is being used by blood banks to screen potentially contaminated blood products.

—CAT scan may reveal central nervous system lesions or atrophy.

—Blood studies may pinpoint metabolic disturbances.

—Brain biopsy is often necessary for definitive diagnosis.

—Medical management includes antiviral, antifungal, and antibacterial agents. There is no known means of restoring the immune system.

—Focal brain irradiation may be used.

—Interferon, used in some patients with Kaposi's sarcoma, Interleukin-2, and AZT are still experimental therapies.

—Treatment still focuses on the secondary illnesses that take advantage of the weakened immune system.

F. Brain Abscess

—Skull films and CAT scan may help diagnostically.

—An arteriogram may be done.

—A lumbar puncture may show increased opening pressure, elevated white count, elevated protein, and presence of polymorphonuclear cells.

—Antibiotics are often used.

—Surgical excision may be possible if the abscess is well encapsulated.

—The abscess may be aspirated and drained. The sac may be then injected with antimicrobial drugs.

SUGGESTED READINGS

Miller J, Arsenault L: Reye's syndrome. *J Neurosurg Nsg* 15(3): 154–164, 1983.
Minnick A: Cysticercosis: etiology and nursing care. *Neurosci Nsg* 18(3): 135–139, 1986.
Nurse's Clinical Library: *Neurologic Disorders*. Springhouse, Pa. 1984.
Sunder J: AIDS: a neurological nursing challenge. *Top Clin Nurs* 6(2): 67–71, 1984.
U.S. Dept. of Health and Human Services and Public Health Service, *AIDS*: Information/ Education Plan to Prevent and Control AIDS in the United States, March 1987, U.S. Gov't Printing Office.

CHAPTER 10

Guillain-Barré Syndrome and Myasthenia Gravis

I. DEFINITION AND DISCUSSION

Guillain-Barré syndrome is a paralytic, reversible disease the etiology of which is still unclear, though thought to be autoimmune in nature. It is also called Landry's paralysis, Guillain-Barré-Strohl's syndrome, Landry-Guillain-Barré syndrome, acute febrile polyneuritis, infectious polyneuritis, postinfectious polyneuritis, and acute inflammatory polyradiculopathy.

Myasthenia gravis is a disorder of neuromuscular transmission, thought to be due to an autoimmune response. It is characterized by weakness and abnormal fatigability of voluntary muscles, especially those involved in ocular movements, respiration, facial expression, swallowing, and chewing.

With Guillain-Barré syndrome there may be acute respiratory involvement to the point of needing mechanical ventilation for the patient. Because the paralysis may not ascend as high as to impair the diaphragm, respiratory support is not always necessary, but the extent of paralysis certainly needs to be monitored over the course of the disease.

Myasthenia gravis may result in respiratory complications from aspiration of food, respiratory infections, and acute respiratory failure. Death from this disease is usually from a respiratory problem.

So with both disorders, Guillain-Barré syndrome and myasthenia gravis, there is potential for respiratory alterations. The activity-exercise functional health pattern is altered when there is respiratory impairment. Impaired gas exchange by the respiratory system does not allow for normal mobility (activity, exercise).

II. ETIOLOGY AND PATHOPHYSIOLOGY

A. Guillain-Barré Syndrome

—May occur at any age, but is more frequent between the ages of 30 and 50 years.

—Males and females affected equally.

—Low mortality rate.

—Five per cent of patients have a recurrence.

—Severity of the disease is increased in the very young and the very old.

—Increased incidence during swine flu vaccination program of 1976.

—Etiology still unclear, but an allergic reaction or an autoimmune response is a strong possibility. Figure 10.1 demonstrates the pathologic changes.

—Related to an antecedent infection, especially viral, in 40% of cases. It has been hypothesized that a viral agent may cause production of antibodies which attack the myelin sheath of peripheral nerves, causing demyelination of the nerve roots. This starts a chain reaction of inflammation, edema, and eventually compression of the nerve root.

—Sometimes occurs after immunizations and also in association with malignant diseases such as Hodgkin's disease and others which affect the lymphatic system.

—The occurrence of Guillain-Barré syndrome after immunization of infectious diseases and sometimes in association with diseases of the lymphoid system all suggest an autoimmune etiology.

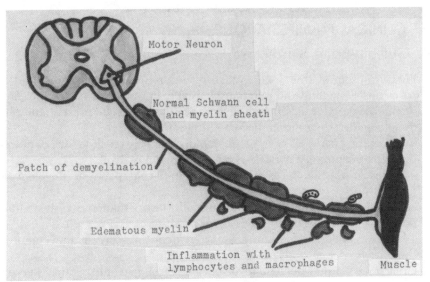

Figure 10.1. Pathologic changes seen in Guillain-Barré syndrome. There is early inflammatory response and edema. Patchy demyelination is a later stage in the disease showing loss of the Schwann cell leaving a widened node of Ranvier. (Reproduced with permission from Prydun M: Guillain-Barré syndrome: disease process. *J Neurosurg Nsg:* 15(1): 29, 1983.)

B. Myasthenia Gravis

—Affects women in their 20s or 30s or men from 40 to 60 years most often. Occurs in females in ratio of 3:1. More black women are victims than white women.

—Incidence is 2–10 persons/100,000. Prevalence is 20,000 to 80,000 cases in the United States.

—Mortality rate is 5–10%, usually due to respiratory paralysis.

—Lower rates of incidence in the southwestern and northern mountain states than in other areas of the United States.

—A transmission disorder at the neuromuscular junction, specifically of the postsynaptic area, thought to be autoimmune in nature.

—There is deactivation of acetylcholine receptor sites, which impairs normal impulse transmission to the muscle. An antiacetylcholine receptor antibody has been demonstrated in most cases of myasthenia gravis.

—Worsens progressively with occasional remissions.

—Respiratory dysfunction results when neuromuscular transmission interferes with respiratory muscle innervation. Gag, swallowing, and cough reflexes, which protect the airway may also be impaired.

—Frequently associated with other autoimmune diseases such as systemic lupus erythematosus, scleroderma, rheumatoid arthritis, pernicious anemia, and Hashimoto's thyroiditis.

III. CLINICAL MANIFESTATIONS

A. Guillain-Barré Syndrome

—First symptom of this degenerative disorder is usually weakness and/or paresthesia (tingling and numbness), usually in the lower extremities, in a symmetrical pattern. Although sensory symptoms may be present, they are usually milder than the motor manifestations.

—An ascending paralysis progressing rapidly that may result in total paralysis, including respiratory paralysis, or may stop at any level.

—No muscle wasting is seen because the flaccid paralysis develops so rapidly.

—Superficial and deep reflexes are usually lost. Cutaneous reflexes (abdominal and cremasteric) are frequently absent.

—Tenderness or pain may be present on deep pressure or movement of the muscle.

—Cranial nerves may become involved. The facial (seventh) cranial nerve is most often affected.

—Autonomic disturbances such as urinary retention and postural hypotension may be seen. Loss of sweating may be present, but in some patients there is an increase in sweating with vasoconstriction, which probably reflects the loss of normal thermal regulation.

—Hypertension may be evident in the acute phase and is associated with an abnormal release of catecholamines.

—Sinus tachycardia and inverted T-waves on electrocardiogram are seen in about 50% of cases.

—Horner's syndrome sometimes occurs.

—Motor function returns in a descending pattern. The rate of remyelinization is about 1–2 mm/day. So the patient's ability to walk returns last.

—Guillain-Barré does not affect level of consciousness, pupillary signs, or cerebral function.

B. Myasthenia Gravis

—Most important clinical sign is weakness of the skeletal muscles, which is relieved by rest and made worse by exercise.

—Muscles supplied by the cranial nerves are most severely involved. Muscles involved in gagging, swallowing, and coughing lose their power to protect the airway. Ptosis and diplopia are common. Loss of facial expression may be evident.

—Proximal muscles of the arms and legs may be affected.

—Respiratory muscles may become too weak to function, leading to acute respiratory failure.

—The ocular form of myasthenia gravis may progress to generalized myasthenia or limit itself to ocular symptoms. Sometimes ocular myasthenia will remit spontaneously.

—Bulbar symptoms may be present, such as dysarthria, dysphagia, and difficulty chewing.

—In severe cases, the bowel and bladder sphincters may be affected, but this is not common.

—Inability to maintain an upward gaze and difficulty with head control may be seen.

—Pupillary signs and cerebral function remain intact.

—Remissions and relapses may occur.

IV. SELECTED MEDICAL PROBLEMS

A. Medical Management

1. Guillain-Barré Syndrome

—Intubation and mechanical ventilation if respiratory musculature is affected.

—Treatment of hypotension or hypertension may be necessary.

—Use of a kinetic bed may be indicated to manage respiratory, autonomic, and musculoskeletal problems.

—Corticosteroids are not routinely used, since they have not been proven to alter the course of the disease.

—Tracheotomy may be done when mechanical ventilation is needed for several weeks.

—The medical management is basically supportive, since there is no specific treatment.

—Nursing care will ultimately determine the clinical course and recovery.

2. Myasthenia Gravis

—Anticholinesterases are used to inhibit the hydrolysis of acetylcholine by acetycholinesterase at the neuromuscular junction. Pyridostigmine bromide (Mestinon) may be the drug of choice due to its long action, fewer side effects, and its stable blood level.

—Thymectomy (surgical excision of the thymus gland) may be performed. It is thought that in some patients this procedure removes a source of antigen and reduces the immune response.

—Corticosteroids may be used in patients with poor response to anticholinesterases and thymectomy. The steroids reduce the amount of antibodies produced via the immune response. Prednisone is often the drug of choice.

—Azothioprine (Imuran) or other immunosuppresive drugs may be used in combination with plasmapheresis.

—Plasmapheresis may be done, whereby circulating antiacetylcholine receptor antibodies in the plasma are removed from the circulation. Symptoms may be relieved for weeks or months in some patients.

—Drugs usually avoided in patients with myasthenia gravis include sedatives, curare, narcotics, antiarrhythmic drugs such as procainamide and quinidine, magnesium sulfate, aminoglycoside and polymixin antibiotics, and quinine. Drugs that may cause hypokalemia, such as steroids and diuretics, may increase muscular weakness.

B. Diagnostic Tests

1. Guillain-Barré Syndrome

—Diagnosis is usually based on the clinical history, clinical manifestations, progression and clinical course. The course is this:
- Acute onset,
- Rapid development of weakness and paralysis,
- Involvement of both the proximal and distal limbs,
- Absence of or only slight muscle atrophy.

—A lumbar puncture may show CSF under normal pressure, an increased CSF protein, without an increase or only a slight increase in white cell count. These findings are not seen initially, but develop several days after onset of symptoms, reaching a peak in 4 to 6 weeks.

—Guillain-Barré is a "rule out" disease. There is no one specific test for it.

—Electromyography (EMG) and nerve conduction velocity tests may be done to rule out other neurologic disorders.

—Pulmonary function tests may be done during the diagnostic workup when

Guillain-Barré is suspected, as a baseline to compare to later pulmonary tests.

2. Myasthenia Gravis

—This disorder may be suspected in patients showing evidence of cranial muscle weakness and progressive muscle fatigue after exertion.

—Thyroid tests, serum creatine phosphokinase, sedimentation rate, and antinuclear antibody levels are usually done.

—A CAT scan of the thymus may be performed.

—The Tensilon (edrophonium chloride) test classically diagnoses the disease. Tensilon is an anticholinesterase. When it is given intravenously, the exhausted muscles are dramatically revived in a patient with myasthenia gravis. Improvement lasts about five minutes. Tensilon is usually used to test the ocular and oropharyngeal muscles. Neostigmine is longer acting, so it is often preferred when evaluating limb strength.

—Tensilon may be used when trying to determine if a patient needs more anticholinesterase or whether he has too much. Myasthenic crisis is when the patient needs more medication. Cholinergic crisis results from an overdose of medication. Tensilon will improve symptoms of a myasthenic crisis. It will exacerbate symptoms of a cholinergic crisis but for only a few minutes. Atropine, a cholinergic reactivator, is given for a cholinergic crisis. Neostigmine may be given for myasthenic crisis.

—Electromyography and nerve conduction tests may help confirm the diagnosis.

SUGGESTED READINGS

Nursing '84 Books, *Neurologic Disorders*. Springhouse, PA, Springhouse, 1984.

Prydun M: Guillain-Barré syndrome: disease process. *J Neurosurg Nsg* 15(1): 27–32, 1983.

Rudy E: *Advanced Neurological, and Neurosurgical Nursing*. St. Louis, CV Mosby, 1984.

Snyder M: *A Guide to Neurological and Neurosurgical Nursing*, New York, John Wiley & Sons, 1983.

Tikkanen P: Landry-Guillain-Barré-Strohl syndrome. *J Neurosurg Nsg:* 14(2): 74–81, 1982.

Hydrocephalus

I. DEFINITION AND DISCUSSION

Hydrocephalus is a clinical syndrome of excessive cerebrospinal fluid (CSF) within the ventricular system that causes the ventricles to dilate. This excessive accumulation of CSF is a result of an imbalance between the production and the absorption of the fluid. When there is excessive CSF accumulation, there is a potential for altered cerebral tissue perfusion due to the increased intracranial pressure. The increased intracranial pressure usually causes an altered mental state. If the hydrocephalus with its concurrent increased intracranial pressure persists within the cranial vault, there is potential for herniation and death of cerebral tissue.

II. GENERAL INFORMATION

A. Etiology

1. Congenital

—Three times more common than acquired hydrocephalus.

—Hydrocephalus ranks third in frequency among major congenital malformations.

—Congenital neoplasm.

—Intrauterine infection.

—Congenital malformation.

  • Arnold-Chiari malformation is one in which there is downward displacement of the fourth ventricle and medulla and obliteration of the cisterna magna by adhesions.

  • Aqueductal stenosis is usually not a complete stenosis, but a forking of, usually, the aqueduct of Sylvius between the third and fourth ventricles into distinct channels separated by normal tissue. Stenosis of the foramina of Luschka and/or Magendie may also occur (Dandy-Walker syndrome).

—Congenital cysts may obstruct flow of CSF or cause hydrocephalus by progressive enlargement.

2. Acquired
—Inflammation.
- Intracranial hemorrhage may cause the meninges to become thickened and fibrosed. When hemorrhage occurs in children with an immature ventricular system, the blood may not be able to be resorbed.
- Infection, such as bacterial meningitis, may produce purulent exudates that obstruct resorption of CSF and cause meningeal thickening from scar tissue formation.

—Neoplasm may obstruct the ventricular system if within the system, or compress the ventricles from an extraventricular mass.
—Trauma may create an obstructive problem as well as a resorption problem.

B. Types of Hydrocephalus

1. Noncommunicating or obstructive hydrocephalus
—Involves an obstruction to the natural flow of CSF.
—Seventy per cent of CSF is made by the choroid plexus in the lateral ventricles. Some is also produced in the third ventricle and the brain parenchyma.
—The flow from the lateral ventricles proceeds into the third ventricle through the foramen of Monro. (Fig. 11.1) It then moves through the aqueduct of Sylvius into the fourth ventricle in the posterior fossa. Two channels allow escape of CSF from the fourth ventricle, the foramen of Luschka and the foramen of Magendie. The CSF then flows into the subarachnoid space bathing the brain and spinal cord. It is then resorbed by arachnoid villi in the dural sinuses.
—Noncommunicating hydrocephalus most frequently results from obstruction of the aqueduct of Sylvius or the foramina of Luschka or Magendie.
—Signs and symptoms include those of increased intracranial pressure (see Chapter 2).

2. Communicating Hydrocephalus
—A problem of impaired resorption or, more rarely, a problem of overproduction of CSF.
—Hemorrhage or particulate matter from infection may occlude the arachnoid villi, hampering resorption.
—Overproduction of CSF may occur in presence of a tumor or hypertrophy of the choroid plexus. Resorption of CSF occurs three to four times as rapidly as it is produced, so overproduction is not commonly seen.
—Signs and symptoms include those of increased intracranial pressure (see Chapter 2).

3. Normal-pressure Hydrocephalus
—Also called occult hydrocephalus, low-pressure hydrocephalus, hydrocephalic dementia, or normotensive hydrocephalus.

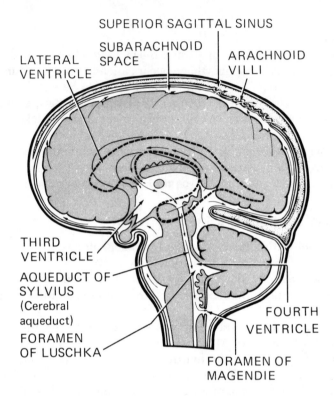

SUPERIOR SAGITTAL SINUS

SUBARACHNOID
SPACE

LATERAL
VENTRICLE

ARACHNOID
VILLI

THIRD
VENTRICLE

AQUEDUCT OF
SYLVIUS
(Cerebral
aqueduct)

FORAMEN
OF LUSCHKA

FOURTH
VENTRICLE

FORAMEN OF
MAGENDIE

Figure 11.1.   Ventricular system and CSF flow. (Reproduced with permission from Snyder, M, Jackle M: *Neurologic Problems*. Norwalk, CT, Appleton-Century-Crofts, 1981, p. 23.)

—It may be the consequence of an old head injury in which there was subarachnoid bleeding or inflammation of the subarachnoid space with scar formation and eventual partial obstruction to the flow of CSF. It may also be a result of thrombosis of the superior sagittal sinus.

—There is ventricular enlargement, but the CSF pressure is normal or near normal when a lumbar puncture is done.

—This is potentially a reversible condition if identified and treated early.

—Signs and symptoms appear slowly. Some signs may be mistakenly attributed to old age in the elderly.

—Cardinal symptoms include mental status changes beginning with forgetfulness and inability to participate in normal conversation, gait disturbances and, later, urinary incontinence.

—Seizures may be evident.

—Nystagmus may be present.

—Lower extemity tendon reflexes may be increased.

—Headache and papilledema and clear cerebellar signs are usually not present.

C. Pathophysiology of Hydrocephalus

—Starling's forces governing fluid transport at the capillary bed level are important to understand (Fig. 11.2). There are definite relationships between filtration and resorption. Formation and resorption of CSF are controlled by the same hydrostatic and colloid osmotic forces that regulate movement of fluid and small particles between the plasma and interstitial fluid compartments of the body.

—Hydrostatic pressure is the force with which fluid presses against the inside of the vessel wall. It is higher at the arterial end of a capillary than at the venous end. It can be thought of as a pushing away force, primarily of water.

—Colloid oncotic pressure (COP) is a water-attracting force. It attracts water into the capillary through the capillary wall. Protein and large molecules make up this osmotic force. These substances are too large to pass across

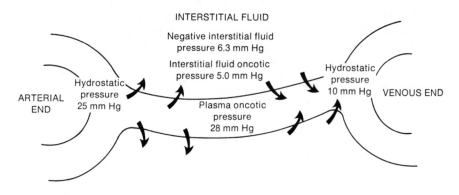

Forces favoring movement out of the capillary		Forces favoring movement into the capillary	
Hydrostatic pressure	25 mm Hg	Plasma oncotic pressure	28 mm Hg
Interstitial pressures	11.3 mm Hg	TOTAL	28 mm Hg
TOTAL	36.3 mm Hg		
Forces favoring movement into the capillary		Forces favoring movement out of the capillary	
Plasma oncotic pressure	28 mm Hg	Hydrostatic pressure	10 mm Hg
TOTAL	28 mm Hg	Interstitial pressures	11.3 mm Hg
		TOTAL	21.3 mm Hg
NET FILTRATION PRESSURE	8.3 mm Hg	NET REABSORPTION PRESSURE	6.7 mm Hg

Figure 11.2. Capillary bed, illustrating effect of Starling's forces governing movement of fluid between intravascular and interstitial compartments (values shown are arbitrary). (Reproduced with permission from Groer M, Shekleton M: *Basic Pathophysiology*, St. Louis, CV Mosby, 1979, p. 260.)

the capillary membrane, so they stay within the vessel. COP is greater at the venous end of the capillary. It favors movement of water from the CSF into the plasma.

—As a result of these pressures and concentration differences on either side of the capillary membrane, fluid moves out of the capillary into the interstitial space at the arterial end of the capillary and is resorbed at the venous end (carrying cellular waste products into the intravascular compartment) (Fig. 11.2). Alteration of any of these forces will alter normal filtration—absorption of fluid.

—The flow of CSF in the ventricles normally reduces CSF hydrostatic pressure, so there is movement of water and small particles from the plasma into the ventricles. The low plasma hydrostatic pressure of blood in the venous sinuses next to the arachnoid villi favors movement of water and solute from the CSF back into the bloodstream.

—Decreased resorption of CSF with consequent development of hydrocephalus results if the CSF osmotic pressure changes. This pressure could increase if excess protein, such as infection, is present in the CSF (bacteria are protein), or if there is excess glucose in the CSF, or if there is breakup of a cerebral thrombus.

—Decreased resorption may result from an increase in hydrostatic pressure also. This may be seen in a patient with hypertension.

—The rate of CSF formation is independent of the intraventricular pressure, but absorption is proportionate to pressure (Fig. 11.3). Below a pressure of approximately 68 mm CSF, absorption ceases.

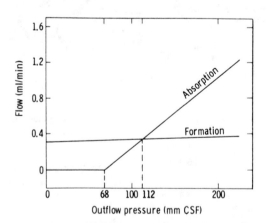

Figure 11.3. CSF formation and absorption in humans at various CSF pressures. Note that at 112 mm CSF, formation and absorption are equal, and at 68 mm CSF, absorption is zero. (Modified and reproduced with permission from Cutler RWP & others: Formation and absorption of cerebrospinal fluid in man. *Brain* 91:707, 1968.)

—Fluid accumulates when the resorption capacity of the arachnoid villi is decreased, as in communicating hydrocephalus. Fluid also accumulates proximal to the block when the foramina of Luschka and Magendie or the aqueduct of Sylvius are occluded (noncommunicating hydrocephalus).

III. GENERAL TREATMENTS

A. Diagnostic Tests

—CAT scan is done to demonstrate presence of enlarged ventricles and enlarged subarachnoid space and site of possible obstruction to CSF flow (Fig. 11.4). It would also reveal a possible mass, such as a tumor, compressing part of the ventricular system, and cortical size and thickness. Hydrocephalus may be monitored by serial CAT scans to determine the effectiveness of the treatment.
—A lumbar puncture may be done if there is no evidence of a mass lesion on CAT scan, so the CSF may be sampled for analysis.
—Radioactive isotope cisternography may be done to demonstrate the flow of CSF. A radioactive isotope is introduced into the cisternal or lumbar sub-

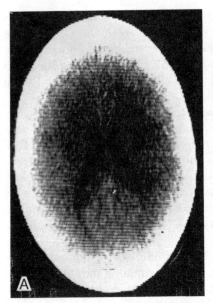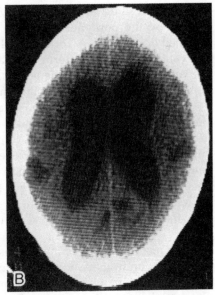

Figure 11.4.   Computerized Tomographic Scans of Lateral Ventricles. *A* Normal sized lateral ventricles. *B* Dilated lateral ventricles seen with obstructive hydrocephalus. (Reproduced by permission from Earnest MP: *Neurologic Emergencies.* New York, Churchill Livingstone, 1983, p. 67.)

arachnoid space. It should flow up to the parasagittal area with little or no intraventricular uptake. If communicating hydrocephalus is present there will be a pattern of prolonged intraventricular concentration of the isotope.

—Pneumoencephalogram is not done as frequently since the advent of the CAT scan, but it can reveal the site of CSF obstruction as well as ventricular enlargement. In patients with normal-pressure hydrocephalus, the air injected into the ventricles rapidly fills them, but there is diminished movement of air into the cerebral subarachnoid space because of the problem with resorption.

—Skull x-rays are not always necessary, but do show thinning of the skull with separation of the sutures and widening of the fontanels in infants.

—Transillumination of the skull may be done in an infant to show fluid accumulation.

—In children with open fontanels, ultrasonography may reveal ventricular dilatation.

—An arteriogram will show enlarged ventricles and vascular displacement.

B. Medical Management

—External ventricular drainage through a ventriculostomy may be used to relieve hydrocephalus temporarily.

—A permanent shunt may be necessary between one of the lateral ventricles and, often, the peritoneal cavity (a V-P shunt) where the CSF can be resorbed or excreted. A Torkildsen shunt is one established between a lateral ventricle and the cisterna magna. The CSF can thus be resorbed into the venous sinuses. A ventriculoatrial shunt allows CSF flow to go from a lateral ventricle into the right atrium.

Most shunts consist of a primary catheter, a reservoir, a one-way valve, and a terminal catheter. The primary catheter is implanted in a lateral ventricle so CSF can flow from the ventricle into the reservoir. As the CSF enters the terminal catheter, it passes through a one-way valve that prevents fluid from refluxing back into the ventricle. The reservoir is close enough to the scalp so that CSF can be withdrawn from it if necessary for analysis or for rapid reduction of intracranial pressure. The terminal catheter leads to the peritoneal cavity, the heart, or the internal jugular vein.

The most common complications from an implanted shunt are infection, occlusion from tissue or exudate, or dislodgment of part of the shunt system. The mortality rate from shunt complications is about 7.2%.

—Cerebral dehydrating agents, such as Mannitol, may be used to control intracranial pressure (see Chapter 2).

—Surgical widening of the foramen magnum may decompress an Arnold-Chiari deformity.

—Surgical removal of a mass, tumor, or cyst may correct the flow of CSF in obstructive hydrocephalus.

—Experimental treatment of hydrocephalus includes the development of valves that regulate CSF flow and open when a preset volume is present. This is different from the more commonly used pressure-regulated valves. The goal is to decrease the likelihood of debris and protein collecting around the valve and obstructing it.

—Drug research is being performed also, in an attempt to develop an agent that may decrease production of CSF. Carbonic anhydrase inhibitors, such as acetazolamide (Diamox), decrease intraventricular production of CSF as much as 50% in animals, but the action is of short duration.

—Cardiac glycosides, such as Oubain and Bromacetyl-Cymarin, inhibit secretion of CSF, but may induce cardiovascular complications.

SUGGESTED READINGS

Arsenault L: Delayed onset symptomatic hydrocephalus related to aqueductal stenosis. *J Neurosurg Nsg* 15(5):291–298, 1983.

Grant L: Hydrocephalus: an overview and update. *J Neurosurg* 16(6):313–318, 1984.

Hickey J: *Clinical Practice of Neurological and Neurosurgical Nursing.* Philadelphia, JB Lippincott, 1981.

Nursing 84 Books, *Neurologic Disorders.* Springhouse, PA, Springhouse, 1984.

CHAPTER 12

Neurologic Disorders Resulting in Dementia

I. DEFINITION AND DISCUSSION

There are numerous conditions that can result in dementia. A few will be discussed in this chapter. Dementia in general is characterized by impairment in mental capacity. Intellectual function, including problem-solving ability, is impaired. Memory, orientation, ability to take in and assimilate new information, and interpretation of the surroundings may all be affected.

There is some nerve cell degeneration in all dementia. That degeneration may result from different mechanisms of injury, such as inflammation, compression, or a biochemical derangement. Whatever the etiology of the dementia, it has a severe impact on both the patient and the family.

The role-relationship functional health pattern is affected because the victim of dementia is unable to perform in his previous role in the family. The spouse, sibling, or child of the demented individual may be forced to become the controller of the finances, the physical caregiver, and the decision-maker. Some or all of these roles may have previously been held by the patient. But roles within the family must be altered to accomodate an individual with dementia.

Dementia is a general term that refers to a progressive global decline in cognitive abilities. This decline eventually impairs attention, memory, judgment, and insight. Affect is also influenced, and personal and social interactions decline along with cognition. How a specific form of dementia presents and how it progresses may be different for different types of dementia. The onset and progression may be fast or slow.

Organic brain syndrome, until recently, was a term used to refer to memory-impaired behavior when no specific cause for the behavior could be found. It was a catch-all term referring to many dementing diseases which cause organic changes in the brain. Senile dementia is a newer term used to describe confused, disoriented, intellectually slow, and memory-impaired patients over the age of 65 years. We now know that senile dementia may be caused by a reversible condition or by an irreversible condition. When the term senile dementia is used to refer to mental changes in the elderly, it is probably a misnomer. We now know that old age in itself does not result in dementia, although the aging brain may be less resistant to diseases that cause dementia.

Presenile dementia is a term sometimes used to refer to the same dementing process seen in senile dementia, but it occurs in patients younger than 65 years of age.

II. ETIOLOGY

A. General Information

Dementia affects approximately 10-15% of the U.S. population over 65 years of age. This means that there are over 1 million people totally dependent for their care, and another 2 million with less severe mental impairment. Fifty to 60% of nursing home residents have dementia. The cost of their care is over $17 billion per year. Our older population is increasing. Those over 65 years of age in the U.S. in 1981 were 11% of the total population. Over the next fifty years, the over-65 population will increase to 20%. In view of these statistics, the potential burden to society for the care of the elderly with dementia is staggering.

Dementia may be a result of many many disorders, some reversible and some non-reversible. Some researchers classify the dementing diseases as follows:

1. Dementia associated with other medical conditions, such as hypothyroidism, Cushing's syndrome, and nutritional deficiencies.
2. Dementia associated with other neurologic signs, such as Huntington's chorea, Creutzfeldt-Jakob disease, brain tumor or trauma.
3. Dementia that is the primary symptom, such as in Alzheimer's or Pick's disease.

Table 12.1 gives an extensive list of etiological factors for dementia.

B. Pathophysiology

1. Alzheimer's Disease

—The most common cause of adult-onset dementia. Comprises 50-70% of all dementias. Approximately 15% of the population over 65 years of age is affected with Alzheimer's and 5% of this group is severely demented.
—Insidious onset.
—Patients are aware of their diminishing intellectual abilities early in the disease.
—Hallmarks of the disease are presence of fibrillary tangles of the neurons (preventing tramsmission of impulses) and neuritic (senile) plaques at the

Table 12.1.
Diseases Causing Dementia*

Diffuse Parenchymatous Diseases of
the Central Nervous System
  So-called presenile dementias
    Alzhemier's disease
    Pick's disease
    Kraepelin's disease
    Parkinsonism-dementia complex
      of Guam
    Huntington's chorea
  Senile dementia
  Other degenerative diseases
    Hallervorden-Spatz disease
    Spinocerebellar degenerations
    Progressive myoclonus epilepsy
    Progressive supranuclear palsy
    Parkinson's disease

Metabolic Disorders
  Myxedema
  Disorders of the parathyroid glands
  Wilson's disease
  Liver disease
  Hypoglycemia
  Remote effects of carcinoma
  Cushing's syndrome
  Hypopituitarism
  Uremia
  Dialysis dementia
  Metachromatic leukodystrophy

Vascular Disorders
  Arteriosclerosis
  Inflammatory disease of blood
      vessels
    Disseminated lupus erythematosus
    Thromboangitis obliterans
    Aortic arch syndrome
    Binswanger's disease
    Arteriovenous malformations

Hypoxia and Anoxia

Normal Pressure Hydrocephalus

Deficiency Diseases
  Wernicke-Korsakoff syndrome
  Pellagra
  Marchiafava-Bignami disease
  Vitamin B_{12} and folate deficiency

Toxins and Drugs
  Metals
  Organic compounds
  Carbon monoxide
  Drugs

Brain Tumors

Trauma
  Open and closed head injuries
  Punch-drunk syndrome
  Subdural hematoma
  Heat stroke

Infections
  Brain abscess
  Bacterial meningitis
  Fungal meningitis
  Encephalitis
  Subacute sclerosing
      panencephalitis
  Progressive multifocal
      leukoencephalopathy
  Creutzfeld-Jakob disease
  Kuru
  Behet's syndrome
  Leu's

Other Diseases
  Multiple Sclerosis
  Muscular Dystrophy
  Whipple's disease
  Concentration-camp syndrome
  Kufs' disease
  Familial calcification of basal
      ganglia

*Reproduced with permission from Haase GR: Diseases presenting as dementia.
In: Well CE (ed): *Dementia*. Philadelphia, FA Davis, 1977, pp. 27–28.
Source: Boss BJ: The dementias. *J Neurosurg Nsg* 15:89, 1983.

synapses between cells in the cortex. The plaques are degenerated cell structures that affect nerve impulse conduction between cells. There are also granulovascular changes: the cells become engorged with fluid-filled vacuoles and granular material.
—Abnormal cellular metabolism, the impairment in transfer of substances between cells, and the displacement of normal cells in the cytoplasm all contribute to memory deficit.
—Brain atrophy results, ventricles enlarge, and sulci widen.
—Theories of etiology include:
  • A deficiency of the enzyme choline acetyltransferase, which is necessary for the production of the neurotransmitter acetylcholine.
  • Increased deposits of aluminum in the brain.
  • Heredity. Patients with Down's syndrome show the same brain pathology as do victims of Alzheimer's disease if they live into their 30s or 40s.
  • Long-term stress may affect the endocrine, immune, and nervous systems, perhaps playing a role in the onset of Alzheimer's disease.
  • Previous severe head trauma has been suggested in some studies to be a precipitating factor in later development of Alzheimer's.
—Four phases of Alzheimer's disease follow although everyone with the disease may not progress through all components of each phase:
  a. Early phase
     —Gradual, subtle manifestations may be seen, such as the patient having less energy and initiative, slower reactions, and being slower at learning new information.
     —Major intellectual deficits may not be perceptible.
     —Short-term memory loss is a cardinal early sign, and the most common early manifestation.
     —There may be mild personality and emotional changes, social withdrawal, irritability, somatic complaints, apraxia, and language disturbances.
  b. Second phase
     —Speech slows.
     —Obvious loss of recent memory; short attention span.
     —Altered sleep patterns.
     —Personal appearance often neglected.
     —May be unable to calculate and need help balancing the checkbook.
  c. Third Phase
     —Disoriented to time, place, and may not be able to identify familiar people.
     —Maladaptive mechanisms may be used to cover up intellectual deficits, such as blaming others, confabulation, and denial.
     —May perseverate, that is, repeat the same action over and over.
     —Inappropriate affect.

—Loss of insight.
—Wandering and losing way.
  d. *Fourth Phase*
    —Apathetic.
    —May need help with most activities of daily living (ADL); loss of motor control.
    —Wandering is more prevalent.
    —May forget to eat.
    —Speech may be unintelligible or mute.
    —Incontinent of urine and/or stool.
    —Gradually becomes weak, uncoordinated, and may become bed-ridden.
    —Does not recognize himself in mirror nor other people.
    —Depression, delusions or delirium may occur.

2. Multiinfarct Dementia (MID)
—MID afflicts 15% of all victims of organic brain disease. Combined with Alzheimer's disease, the two classes account for about 90% of all dementia.
—Usually occurs between ages of 40 and 60 years.
—Predisposing factor is cardiovascular arteriosclerosis. Hypertension, diabetes, obesity, heart attacks, angina, and cigarette smoking have all been associated with MID.
—Cognitive loss has an abrupt onset, accompanied by focal signs of the precipitating vascular event.
—Dementia resulting from MID is similar to that resulting from cerebral atrophy.
—Pathology consists of multiple small areas of infarction in the cortex or underlying white matter or several major strokes involving both hemispheres.
—Greater preservation of memory than other cognitive abilities, especially speech.
—Focal neurologic deficit is evident.
—Decline in mental ability is stepwise rather than gradual, due to repeated strokes. There may be a remission to near normal mental functioning and emotional affect in early stages.
—Pseudobulbar palsy may be present, which is not present in Alzheimer's.

3. Parkinsonian Dementia
—Ten to 20% of those with Parkinson's disease develop dementia, usually late in the illness.
—Cognition and social behavior are affected.
—Dementia results in:
  • Impaired problem solving.
  • Poor judgment; lack of insight.
  • Lack of social graces.

- Difficulty with concept formation.
- General apathy.

—Some researchers believe that antiparkinsonism drugs produce changes in reasoning and accentuate the severity of any underlying dementia.

—Others believe that dementia is related to the severity of the Parkinson's disease.

—Some researchers believe there are two forms of parkinsonism, one characterized by tremor with intact intellectual ability, and another characterized by akinesia and neuropsychological deficits.

—Still others believe dementia seen in parkinsonian patients is a result of coexistence with Alzheimer's disease. The subcortical changes are due to the Parkinson's disease, and the cortical changes due to Alzheimer's.

4. Multiple Sclerosis Dementia

—Occurs late in the disease due to extensive cerebral demyelination.

—Characterized by euphoria, irritability, emotional instability, and depression.

—Cognitive deficits may not be pronounced, but focus on inability to utilize new information.

5. Huntington's Disease

—Huntington's disease is a genetic disorder characterized by choreiform movements and mental deterioration. The intellectual deficits are more incapacitating than the movement disorder.

—Poor judgment may precede clear intellectual deterioration.

—Dementia usually occurs late in the disease, with memory and cognitive deficits.

—Initially, changes in emotional and social behavior are seen.

—Apathy, mood swings, violent temper, inattention to personal grooming may all appear.

—Keenly aware of their intellectual deterioration in the early stages.

—Cellular loss is most extensive in the putamen and caudate nucleus.

—Levels of glutamic acid decarboxylase, which is necessary for synthesis of gamma-aminobutyric acid (the inhibitory transmitter substance), and levels of choline are significantly low in the caudate nucleus.

—There are fewer than normal number of receptor binding sites for serotonin and muscarinic acetylcholine with Huntington's disease.

—Like Alzheimer's disease and parkinsonism, there is a disruption of neurotransmission. Like parkinsonism, this disease involves mostly the subcortical structures, although there is also some destruction of cortical cells.

6. Pick's Disease

—Characteristic nerve cell changes are concentrated in the frontal and temporal lobes, rather than the generalized changes and atrophy seen with Alzheimer's.

—Average age of onset is 40–50 years of age.

—Cognition is spared in early stages, but changes in personality and behavior are apparent, such as loss of inhibition and social graces.

—Patients have no insight into their behavioral deterioration.

—Cognitive impairment, as the disease progresses, resembles that of Alzheimer's disease.

—In second stage of dementia, there is loss of facial expression and language deficits (anomia and scanty speech production and eventually loss of comprehension of speech). Perseveration and echolalia may be evident. If apraxias occur, they are less severe than those seen in Alzheimer's victims.

—In the final stage, dementia is profound, resembling an advanced Alzheimer's patient; passive, vegetative behavior with little or no memory.

7. Creutzfeldt-Jakob Disease

—Disease is due to a transmissible virus that produces a spongiform encephalopathy; rapidly progressing disease resulting in death.

—Myoclonic jerks, ataxia or rigidity accompany the dementia.

—Changes in mental status often begin with confusion. Psychosis may result. These changes progress to dementia and to a state of akinetic mutism and rigidity, coma, and death within 6 months to 2 years.

—Neurons are absent and gliosis is severe with spongy breakdown of brain substance.

III. GENERAL TREATMENTS

A. Diagnostic Tests

The most important differential diagnosis is distinguishing dementia (from whatever cause) from depression. Depression may look like dementia clinically, that is, a depressed person may demonstrate anxiety and agitation, have a low self-esteem, and move and speak slowly. Depressed patients appear to have memory gaps and intellectual impairment. Family history of depression is significant in the diagnosis, and if the depressed patient is treated with antidepressants, he most often improves. Antidepressants do not change the behavior of a demented person. Other clinical clues in differentiating similar disorders are shown in Table 12.2.

1. Alzheimer's Dementia

—Brain biopsy is the only sure way to diagnose Alzheimer's. Evidence of neurofibrillary tangles and plaques with positive fuchsin staining will be found.

—CAT scan shows brain atrophy and usually enlarged ventricles. It helps rule out many other disorders.

—PET scan shows areas of brain affected by Alzheimer's disease use less oxygen than the normal brain. (Fig. 12.1)

—EEG shows a diffuse slowing of electrical activity in most patients.

Table 12.2.
Differential Diagnosis of Dementia

Cause	Clinical clues	Confirmatory tests
Alzheimer's disease	No other neurologic signs	CT scan
Pick's disease	Symptoms less global then Alzheimer's	CT scan
Multi-infarct dementia	Pseudobulbar palsy; episodic worsening	CT scan may show lacunar infarcts
Depression	Depressed mood	Response to anti-depressants
Drugs (tranquilizers, antiparkinsonian agents)	History of drug use; slurred speech, ataxia, lethargy, withdrawal symptoms or improve-ment in hospital	Toxicology screen
Chronic subdural hematoma	History of drinking, anticoagulant therapy, lethargy, headache	CT scan, brain scan
B_{12} deficiency	Ataxia, posterior column signs	CBC, B_{12} level, Schilling test
Hydrocephalus	Incontinence, gait disturbance	CT scan, isotope cisternography
Hypothyroidism	Husky voice, stiff muscles, "hung up" reflexes	Thyroid studies
Syphilis	Tongue tremor, miotic pupils	VDRL, FTA
Chronic meningitis (fungus, tumor, tuberculosis)	Other signs of systemic disease	LP for cells, glucose, cytology
Huntington's disease	Parent or siblings in mental hospital; fidgety on physical exam	CT scan for caudate atrophy
Creutzfeldt-Jakob disease	Progression over months; myoclonus	EEG: triphasic sharp waves

CBC, complete blood count; *VDRL,* Veneral Disease Research Laboratories; *FTA,* fluorescent treponemal antibody test; *LP,* lumbar puncture. (Reproduced with permission from Swanson PD (ed): *Signs and Symptoms in Neurology.* Phildelphia, JB Lippincott, 1984, p. 18.)

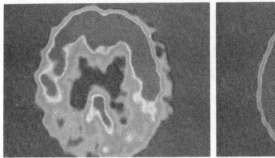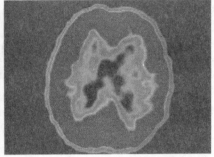

Figure 12.1. A PET scan of a normal brain, right, is in dramatic contrast to one of a patient with Alzheimer's disease. (Reproduced with permission from Restak R: *The Brain.* 1984, Bantam Books, New York, p 340.)

—Lumbar puncture may rule out infections, malignancies, and neurosyphilis.
—Blood tests may rule out treatable causes of dementia, such as thyroid, kidney, and liver abnormalities, nutritional deficiencies, some infections and metabolic imbalances.
—Mental status exam and complete neurologic exam will provide a baseline status.
—Pneumoencephalogram often shows frontal and temporal lobe atrophy.
—Nuclear magnetic resonance scanning may be helpful in ruling out many treatable causes of dementia.

2. Multiinfarct Dementia
—History is very important if it includes past small "strokes."
—Signs and symptoms of vascular disease should be searched for, rather than performance on mental status exams. Check for precipitating factors, such as hypertension.

3. Parkinsonian Dementia
—CAT scan may show dilated ventricles and diffuse cortical atrophy.
—EEG shows diffuse slowing of theta waves.

4. Multiple Sclerosis Dementia
—CAT scan shows increased tissue density of white matter.
—EEG may show nonspecific changes in some patients.

5. Huntington's Dementia
—CAT scan shows caudate atrophy and usually enlarged ventricles.
—EEG often shows loss and slowing of alpha activity.

6. Pick's Dementia
—CAT scan may show focal loss of brain substance in one or both frontotemporal regions as well as the thalamus and basal ganglia, with a decrease in white matter being more marked than that of gray matter.

7. Creutzfeldt-Jakob Dementia

—CAT scan may show cerebral atrophy late in the disease.
—EEG findings are progressive and eventually diagnostic of the disorder. Initially, there is slowing of background rhythm over both hemispheres. The frequency of these spikes increases and is superimposed on a slow, low voltage background.
—Brain biopsy confirms the diagnosis.

B. Medical Management

—Some trial drugs are being used to treat Alzheimer's dementia, such as hydergine (a vasodilator thought to stimulate cerebral circulation), choline and lecithin (neurotransmitter precursors) and physostigmine, which prevents breakdown of acetylcholine. Propranolol has been used experimentally to treat aggressive behavior in elderly brain-damaged patients. Geronital H-3 has not been shown to enhance memory, but it may have a weak antidepressant effect.

Some drugs given as sedation to patients with Alzheimer's disease, such as haloperidol (Haldol) is an anticholinergic which may make memory worse. Naloxone is used experimentally to improve mental performance and memory. Neuropeptides, such as vasopressin and the hormone ACTH, are also being studied.

—Research is being done on transplanting brain cells from one animal to another. In rats that have diabetes insipidus, provoked by a congenital lack of certain brain cells, transplantation of the missing cells from normal rats often cures the disease. So, theoretically, it may be possible to transplant cholinergic brain cells into the brains of patients with Alzheimer's disease.

—Some physicians think memory training techniques are helpful to slow down the dementia.

—Judicious use of tranquilizers may be necessary to control violent behavior.

—Although the neuronal damage done with MID cannot be reversed, in some cases treatment of underlying conditions such as hypertension, carotid artery stenosis, and cardiac dysrhythmias may stop progression of the dementia.

—Parkinson's disease responds well to L-dopa, a substance needed for production of the neurotransmitter dopamine, which Parkinson's disease patients lack.

—Most dementias have no specific treatment to cure the process. Therapy is directed at maintaining and maximizing use of the available capacities.

—Correction of metabolic systemic disorders is important, since these disturbances can make the mental status worse.

Ten Commandments for Families of Alzheimer's Patients

1. Thou shalt seek legal aid for financial planning soon after diagnosis.
2. Thou shalt not be ashamed of thy patient.
3. Thou shalt not refuse any assistance from relative or friend or neighbor or government.
4. Thou shalt discuss problems with a wise listener.
5. Thou shalt laugh and cry occasionally.
6. Honor thy loved one who is ill and remember that love lasts.
7. Seek out a support group to help with problems.
8. Admit feelings of anger, guilt, or resentment but do not enshrine them.
9. Leave thy patient one day in seven in order that thou be strengthened for the long hard journey ahead.
10. Wear each day as a loose garment. Enjoy a smile, the warm sun, the flash of birds, or the laughter of a child.

Shall We Laugh or Cry?

As the years pass, my husband and I grow less and less able to communicate. He is a victim of Alzheimer's Disease, a malady which slowly renders brain cells useless, an illness that strikes at the very heart of our humanness. As his world dwindles, I feel frustrated as I try to talk to him but I sense his response to a guiding hand, a loving touch, or a smile.

Today I long to share my delight with him so I bring our two small newly-adopted granddaughters to visit him in a nursing home nearby. Pleased, I watch their little hands pat and hug him.

Together, we tug grandpa out of his geriatric chair to take him for a walk. Suddenly I realize that I don't have enough arms to go down the stairs with a two-year old, a three-year old, and an agile patient with the mind of a two-year old. I'd better take the elevator. The doors slide open and soon everyone is herded inside. I see the panic start in the eyes of both girls as the new experience startles them. I kneel down quickly and place a reassuring arm around each. Grandpa watches and mimics my act of kneeling and hugging. The tiny girls blink solemnly and they kneel too.

When the elevator opens, a nurse looks down on our strange circle. Then we all begin laughing in glee—each for his own reason—and for one moment our worlds merge.

Figure 12.2. "Ten Commandments for Families of Alzheimer's Patients" (compiled by North Shore Support Group) and "Shall We Laugh or Cry?" are from a 1987 newsletter published by ADRDA (Alzheimer's Disease and Related Disorders Association).

13

Acute and Chronic Pain

I. DEFINITION AND DISCUSSION

Pain is a subjective experience. It is often categorized by its expected duration. Pain management is modified according to the cause of the pain. Acute pain usually refers to a relatively sudden onset and pain of limited duration, due to an obvious injury or disease state. It often is lifesaving, such as initiating restrictive or withdrawal behavior. Examples of acute pain include postoperative incisional pain, myocardial infarction, fractured bones, and needle pricks. Acute pain may last from seconds up to weeks or months, but it is self-limiting. Intensity of acute pain is usually an indicator of the severity of the injury or disease. It acts as a warning that something may be wrong. Acute pain is accompanied by autonomic responses, such as tachycardia, hypertension,

Gate-control Theory of Pain

This theory proposed by Melzack and Wall suggest that neural mechanisms in the dorsal horns of the spinal cord function as gates that can open or close to the flow of nerve impulses from peripheral fibers to the central nervous system. In this manner, there is control of pain signals entering the central pain pathways. The theory proposes that stimulation of the large (fast) A fibers decreases the effectiveness of the small (slow) fibers in transmitting pain messages. The fast fibers receive peripheral stimuli as well as stimuli from the cortex, brainstem, and limbic area, thus modifying the emotional response. When the large fibers are stimulated by nonpainful stimuli such as heat or touch, the pain input is blocked and the gate is closed, so pain is relieved.

Skeletal muscle activity, such as exercise, produces inhibition of the small fiber pain system. It is thought that this is due to the high amount of large A fiber traffic during exercise. Thus exercise is often a recommended part of the management regime for chronic pain.

Heat impulse traffic coming into the area of the substantia gelatinosa on the large A fiber sensory system seems to depress conduction in the synapses of the small A delta and C fiber sensory system that relay pain impulses. The converse is also true. When there are incoming impulses on the small fiber network to open the gates, pain is perceived.

diaphoresis, decreased urinary output, and slowing of peristalsis. The patient often protects the painful body part.

Chronic pain allows the patient little time when the mind is free from the thought of pain. Pain can go on for months with no predictable time limitation. It is relatively benign pain. The cause may be known but untreatable, or it may be unknown. Examples of chronic pain are low back pain, arthritis pain, phantom limb pain, or neuropathic pain (neuralgia, peripheral neuritis). Chronic pain victims do not demonstrate autonomic signs. They seem to suffer increasingly the longer the pain is present. They often are depressed, tired-looking, and may focus on the pain exlusively in their lives. Under added stress, the intensity of the pain may increase. Regression and dependent behavior may be demonstrated.

Intractable pain is a term often used synonomously with chronic pain. Other authors distinguish it from chronic pain in that it is constant and due to an incurable cause. It progresses rather than diminishes. An example is terminal cancer pain.

Brain Peptides

There are opiate receptors on cell membranes of specific neurons in the brain, brainstem, and spinal cord that mediate the functions of endogenous opiates. Endorphins are neurosecretory substances (that is, produced in the brain) and are capable of occupying the same opiate receptor sites as morphine. It is thought that endorphins relieve pain by affecting the perception of pain, as occurs in morphine and other opiate administration. Some researchers indicate that patients with chronic pain syndromes have depleted endorphins. External influences, such as electrical stimulation or stress, may increase the endorphin level in an individual. This may explain the delayed pain response in patients who have suffered severe injuries, the euphoria and altered pain perception of long-distance runners, and the effectiveness of some nontraditional pain management techniques, such as biofeedback and acupuncture.

There is speculation about the role of endorphins in drug dependency. Some suggest that exogenous opiates bind the receptor sites and, after a period of exogenous narcotics use, the release of endorphins is inhibited, thus increasing dependency on external sources of narcotics, causing withdrawal when the source is removed.

The cognitive-perceptual functional health pattern is influenced by pain. Pain perception is an individual experience. It may be influenced by physical, psychological, and emotional stimuli. Coping mechanisms of individuals for pain vary widely also. So this functional health pattern may be altered greatly or slightly.

The focus of this chapter will be on headache, representing acute pain, and low back pain as being representative of chronic pain.

II. ETIOLOGY AND PATHOPHYSIOLOGY

A. Headache

1. General Information

—Approximately 42 million Americans experiance headache severe enough to seek medical attention each year.

—Along with the temporary discomfort of the headache is often a fear of some underlying disorder such as a brain tumor.

—The skull (except the periosteum), brain parenchyma, most of the dura, and the ependymal lining of the ventricles are largely insensitive to pain.

—Extracranial tissues of the head are pain-sensitive. This includes the skin, scalp, muscle, arteries, veins, cranial nerves V, VII, IX, X, and the first three cervical nerves.

—Intracranial sources of pain include:

- Dilatation of scalp arteries.
- Traction or displacement of arteries.
- Venous sinuses.
- Compression, traction, or inflammation of sensory or cranial nerves.
- Spasm of cranial or cervical muscles.
- Structural lesions such as brain tumors, subarachnoid hemorrhage, meningitis, arteritis.

2. Classification

a. *Vascular Headaches*

Classic Migraine

- Tends to run in families, often beginning in late childhood or early adolescence.
- Recurrent and periodic.
- Usually preceded by some neurologic warning, premonition, or aura, such as transient blindness, flickering lights, a visual scotoma, hemianopsia, paresis of an extremity, or dysphasia. This neurologic deficit is believed to occur during the vasoconstrictive phase of the headache. Focal areas of ischemia can be produced by the vasospasm. During the second phase, the vasodilatation of extracranial vessels occurs, causing the pain. The neurologic deficit usually precedes the pain by about 15 minutes. Migraine involves vasoconstriction, a vasodilatation, platelet aggregation, and inflammation. One theory is that vascular change may not be the primary event, but rather a peripheral response to a complicated change within the brainstem or hypothalamus. The migraine syndrome is probably a complex network of impairment affecting cognition, appetite or sleep, that develops over several days, with the headache occurring at the peak of the course.
- Onset of the pain is gradual, with increasing intensity.

- Headache is often unilateral (often on the same side as the previous neurologic deficit), and throbbing in nature.
- May be accompanied by nausea and vomiting and/or diarrhea. Photophobia is also common.
- Duration is from several hours to days.
- After the headache there may be a period of muscle contraction of the scalp or neck, causing deep aching and sensitivity to touch.
- Most often begins after awakening, but may begin at any time of the day.

Common Migraine
- Similar to classic headache except with no aura and no neurologic symptoms. Some patients may feel an awareness of a forthcoming headache however.
- May not be a family history of headaches.
- Rarely occur in patients before early adulthood.
- Usually begins with a prodrome of depression or irritability followed by slowly increasing pain.
- Duration is several hours to days.
- May begin during a period of relaxation following a stressful time. May also occur during premenstrual tension and fluid retention. Incidence often decreases during pregnancy.
- Constant and throbbing in nature.
- May be unilateral or bilateral pain.
- May be accompanied by chills, feverishness, depression, fatigue, nausea, vomiting, or nasal congestion.

Complicated Migraine (Hemiplegic and Ophthalmoplegic Forms)
- Recurrent hemiparesis or hemiplegia occurs with the headache (sometimes lasting several days to weeks) or a third nerve palsy. The paralysis usually resolves completely.
- Paralysis is thought to be a result of vasoconstriction in branches of the internal carotid and middle cerebral arteries.
- Ophthalmoplegic migraines usually involve unilateral pain behind or over the eye (frontal or temporal areas). The pain precedes the ocular paralysis, which may appear 6 to 10 hours after the attack of pain. The symptoms may be a result of a dilated and swollen arterial wall exerting pressure on the nerve.
- Occurs most often in young adults.
- Ophthalmoplegic migraines may increase in intensity and frequency during menopause or with the onset of hypertension and vascular disease.

Cluster Headache (Histamine Headache)
- Occurs with a daily attack for several days or weeks. Patient may then be headache-free for several weeks or months before another attack.

- The hypothalamus is believed to be the primary site of cluster headache cycles.
- Usually unilateral pain, of a steady burning or gnawing nature, often occurring at night during REM sleep, lasting an hour or two. Often begins after the patient has been asleep 2 to 3 hours.
- Usually accompanied by signs of parasympathetic overactivity on the affected side, such as tearing, facial flushing or swelling, miosis, ptosis, and enophthalmos. Rhinorrhea or nasal congestion of the side of the headache may also be present.
- Pain is usually in the area of the orbit or in the temporal region.
- More often occurs in older males (male-female ration is 6:1).
- Unlike the patient with a migraine headache who wants to lie still, the patient with a cluster headache often paces, and may even bang his head against a wall or threaten suicide.
- Precipitating factors for increased frequency of attacks during the time a cluster is occurring are emotional upsets, heavy meals, a period of stress or the letdown following the stress, alcohol intake, and use of nitroglycerine or organic nitrates.
- At the onset of a cluster headache the blood level of histamine is said to be elevated. An injection of histamine will precipitate an attack.
- Sometimes there is ipsilateral constriction of pupil if a partial Horner's syndrome develops during the headache.
- Seasons may influence frequency of cluster headaches. Most clusters occur in spring, with fall a close second.

Temporal Arteritis Headache
- Blindness may be present if the central retinal artery is involved.
- The pain is often throbbing or burning in nature, may be unilateral or bilateral, and is centered over the temples.
- Numbness or tenderness of the scalp over the temporal artery is usual.
- Usually occurs in patients over 50 years of age, more often in females than males.
- Etiology is thought to be inflammation of the temporal artery (a branch of the external carotid artery). The artery may appear prominent and tortuous and is rigid and nodular to palpation with diminished pulsation.
- Other symptoms may include fever, confusion, myalgias, arthralgias, fatigue, and focal neurologic deficits.
- Elevated erythrocyte sedimentation rate may help diagnosis of this type of headache.

Hypertensive Headache
- Usually throbbing and continuous in nature, often worse in the morning, and may disappear after the patient has been up and active for an hour or so.

- Paroxysmal.
- Often involves occipital or frontal area of head.
- May be a result of toxemia of pregnancy, malignant hypertension, or end-stage renal disease.
- May be related to hypertensive encephalopathy, so the patient may demonstrate nausea, vomiting, altered level of consciousness, focal neurologic deficits, and seizures.
- Essential hypertension may exacerbate preexisting headaches of other causes.

b. *Some Nonvascular Headaches*

Muscle Contraction Headache (tension headache)
- Pain may be generalized, band-like in the posterior neck, or frontooccipital. Usually originates in occipital area.
- Pain is aggravated by neck motion or postural strain.
- May persist for hours, days or weeks.
- Etiology is sustained muscle contractions, resulting in an accumulation of metabolites. Doesn't involve a permanent structural change.
- May be complicated in the elderly by degenerative joint disease of the cervical spine.
- May be associated with a chronically stressful lifestyle or depression.
- Often begin in afternoon or evening.

Sinus Headache
- Fairly uncommon.
- Dull, deep, aching in nature, aggravated by shaking or tilting the head.
- Usually bilateral, over frontal facial area.
- Face may be tender over sinus area.
- Pain may be worse in the morning, but may be relieved by erect posture, allowing the sinus to drain.
- Nasal tissue may be swollen, nasal congestion, and purulent nasal discharge present. Fever may be evident.
- Transillumination may demonstrate fluid levels.
- Etiology of pain is thought to be inflammation of the nasofrontal ducts and the superior nasal spaces.

Traction or Inflammatory Headache
- Due to traction on or inflammation of intracranial arteries, veins, venous sinuses, or some cranial nerves.
- Common causes of the traction on intracranial structures include hematomas (epidural, subdural, intracerebral), tumors, abscesses, and increased intracranial pressure from conditions such as hydrocephalus or cerebral edema.
- Usually steady, deep and aching in nature. Aggravated by anything which increases intracranial pressure, such as coughing.

- Accompanying symptoms may include nausea, vomiting, a change in level of consciousness or behavior, or cranial nerve signs.

Spinal Tap Headache

- Complication following a lumbar puncture. Usually seen a few hours after lumbar puncture, but may develop a day or two after the procedure.
- Related to posture. When flat in bed, the patient has no headache. When upright the head aches.
- Generalized and bifrontal headache.
- Etiology is a tear or puncture in the dura, allowing cerebrospinal fluid (CSF) to leak into the soft tissue, causing a chronic low cerebrospinal fluid pressure.
- A similar headache may occur after head trauma when a CSF leak has been created due to a skull fracture. The dura is penetrated especially in injuries to the base of the skull (basilar skull fracture) or the cribiform plate, allowing communication into the sinus or the petrous bone with leakage to the middle ear.

3. Medical Management

Treatment (Table 13.1)

—Pain tolerance may vary from individual to individual, and it may vary from time to time with the same individual. Some generalizations about pain tolerance are:

- Women seem to tolerate pain less well than men.
- Older individuals seem to tolerate pain less well than younger individuals.
- The more control an individual feels he has over the pain, the better it is tolerated (for example, relaxation methods, self-regulated medications, etc.).
- High anxiety and denial may be seen in those with less pain tolerance.
- Predictability increases pain tolerance (such as the patient understanding the cause and course).

—Treatment of the acute attack is based on the patient's history, and the therapy that works best for him. A trial of several approaches may be helpful before prescribing long-term management.

- Aspirin or other analgesics.
- Ergomar sublingual.
- Sinubid (a vasoconstrictor).
- Oxygen.
- Steroids and methysergide are the drugs of choice in treating cluster headaches. Cluster headaches do not respond well to beta blockers.

—Psychological consultation is appropriate when emotional issues appear to influence chronic headaches.

Table 13.1.
Common Pharmaceutical Products Useful in Migraine: Oral Prophylactic Therapy

Drug	Dosage
Ergotamine tartrate	1 mg twice daily—skip one day a week
Ergotamine, phenobarbital, and belladonna (various strengths)	1 tablet twice or thrice daily
Methysergide maleate	2 mg two to four times daily (given for no more than six months continuously)
Pheneizine sulfate	15 mg three times daily
Cyproheptadine	4–16 mg daily as tolerate
Propranolol	20 mg three times daily (with increase as required to maximum of 240 mg a day)
Amitriptyline	50–100 mg at bedtime
Clonidine	0.1 mg three times daily
Platelet inhibitors	Varied dosages

Calcium channel blockers
  Verapamil
  Nifedipine
	
	80–120 mg three times daily
	10 mg three times daily, increasing to 20 mg three times daily if necessary

(Reproduced with permission from Dalessio, D: Migraine headaches. *Hospital Medicine* March 1985, Hospital Publications Inc. p 242.)

—Steroids begun immediately may offer relief from temporal arteritis headaches.
—Drugs to control nausea, whether from the migraine or as a side effect of ergotamine may be prescribed, such as phenothiazine suppositories or metoclopramide (Reglan).
—Active range of motion of the head through flexion, extension, lateral flexion and rotation may offer some relief with muscle contraction headaches.
—Antidepressants may be useful in treatment of muscle contraction or tension headaches.
—Nonpharmacologic treatment may include ice packs to the head, sleep, or rest in a quiet, darkened room.
—Phenelzine (Nardil) may be used for headaches refractory to more conservative modes of therapy. It is a monoamine oxidase inhibitor.

Headache History
The headache history is essential in assessing a patient for head pain. The history should include the following:

1. Onset—migraines usually have a gradual onset, often after a period of stress, such as on weekends. Onset of migraines is periodic, and they follow a usual course for that individual. Muscle contraction headaches, however, occur sporadically and often worsen during times of stress. Sinus headaches typically begin in the morning.

2. Location—complaint of unilateral headache suggests migraine or organic dysfunction. Pain over an eye suggests a cluster headache or ocular disease. Generalized head pain suggests muscle contraction headache.

3. Duration—migraines last from 6 hours to 3 days or longer. Cluster headaches involve recurring attacks, each lasting less than 90 minutes, and the entire daily episode lasting less than 4 hours. Cluster headaches may be seasonal. Muscle contraction headaches have a less definate duration.

4. Severity—migraine pain is intense, throbbing and incapacitating. Cluster pain may be described as throbbing also, but is often also described as burning, deep, penetrating or unbearable. Muscle contraction headache is dull, continuous, nagging, or a feeling of pressure.

5. Prodrome—the prodrome, or aura, prior to a classic migraine precedes the pain by 10-20 minutes and often includes flashing lights, scotomata, paresthesia, vertigo, and—rarely—olfactory sensations. Common migraine may have a vague undefined prodrome or none at all.

6. Associated Symptoms—descriptions of nausea, vomiting, chills, anorexia, pallor, photophobia, urinary urgency, or aversion to sound may be given by patients with migraines. Patients with cluster pain may describe facial flushing, stuffy nose, tearing, or ptosis. Symptoms often described with muscle contraction headaches include scalp tenderness, anxiety, neck and shoulder cramping. A history of double vision, convulsions, or tinnitus should make the history-taker suspicious of organic disease.

7. Sleeping Habits—sleep often helps relieve migraine headaches. Cluster headaches often occur at night, awakening the patient. Difficulty falling asleep or frequent awakening may suggest depression or psychogenic problems.

8. Precipitating Factors—stress, endocrine factors, dietary factors, eyestrain, intrinsic and extrinsic factors may all contribute to several types of headache, but are more often described in migraines. Inquiry should be made as to whether there has been recent head trauma, and whether the patient works around chemicals or noxious fumes.

9. Menstrual History—women may have "menstrual migraines" with accompanying weight gain and breast enlargement. The headache may occur prior to, during, or following menses. A description of amenorrhea in a premenopausal woman may suggest a prolactin-producing microadenoma.

10. Emotional Factors—as the headache history is being given, the history-taker should be assessing factors that may have emotional significance to the individual. For example, what is his relationship to his family, how is his job, social and sex life, does he have compulsive, perfectionist traits?

11. Family History—migraine sufferers more often have a history of migraines in their family, but patients with muscle contraction headaches may also describe such a family pattern. Cluster headache sufferers do not show a family predisposition.

12. Medication—previous medications that supplied relief from head pain are important. If, for example, antidepressants were previously effective, the headache may have been from muscle contraction. If ergotamine tartrate provided relief, it may have been a migraine. Migraines may be precipitated or aggravated by birth-control pills, nitrates, and reserpine. Current medications being taken by the patient are important, and may be precipitating the pain.

—Dipyridamole (Persantine) acts as a vasodilator and an agent for antiplatelet aggregation. It may reduce prodromal symptoms of a migraine.

—Narcotics such as meperidine or codeine may provide relief once a vascular headache has begun.

—Ergotamine is contrainicated in patients with hypertension. Hypertensive headaches may be reduced by lowering the patient's blood pressure with antihypertensive drugs.

—Propranalol is contrainicated in patients who have bronchospastic lung disorders, congestive heart failure, and cardiac conduction defects and in those receiving hypoglycemic therapy or monoamine oxidase inhibitors. May be used in patients with hypertension, peripheral vascular disease or coronary artery disease.

—In the case of spinal tap headaches or those due to a CSF leak, bedrest is necessary to allow the dura to seal and to keep the CSF pressure normalized. If the CSF leak does not seal spontaneously, surgical closure may be necessary.

Prevention

• Drugs of choice to prevent many vascular headaches are ergotamine tartrate (Cafergot), a vasoconstrictor, propranolol (Inderal), a beta adrenergic blocker, methysergide maleate (Sansert), a vasoconstrictor. The ability to reverse the headache at the vascular level is more advantageous than having the patient take analgesics, which only offer sensory blockade. Midrin (isometheptane mucate/acetaminophen/chloral phenazone) is often as effective as the ergots and often better tolerated.

• Benzodiazepines may be used in migraine prophylaxis, but drug dependency limits their usefulness.

• Biofeedback may be useful for vascular headaches. This technique trains the patient to control his physiologic responses, altering peripheral blood flow, pulse, and blood pressure.

• Identification and subsequent elimination of "trigger factors" from the

patient's lifestyle may help in prevention of vascular headaches (for example, avoidance of alcohol, certain foods or caffeine).
- Nonsteroidal antiinflammatory drugs show promise as abortive agents. They probably work by inhibiting platelet aggregation and prostaglandin synthesis.
- Amitriptyline (Elavil, Endep) is the drug of first choice for prevention of chronic muscle contraction headache.
- Calcium channel blockers block the calcium-mediated vasospasm of the migraine. Especially useful for prevention and/or treatment of classic migraine. Currently showing encouraging results in prevention of chronic cluster headaches.
- Lithium carbonate is effective in preventing cluster headaches.
- Avoidance of alcohol is a most important factor in management of cluster headaches.
- Foods containing tyramine may be omitted from the diet in a program designed to prevent or control vascular headaches. Such foods include chocolate, yogurt, cheese, vinegar and animal organs. Tyramine is thought to influence serotonin and norepinephrine release. Nitrite and monosodium glutamate also may trigger vascular headaches with their vasodilating effect.

4. Diagnostic Tests
—A complete neurologic and physical exam should be done. Special attention should be given to the blood pressure, head, eyes, ears, nose, throat, teeth and neck, signs of depression, pituitary and thyroid deficiencies, "cafe au lait" spots (often associated with intracranial tumors), and signs of local infection and vascular disease. The patient should be checked for systemic diseases since many may be a contraindication for prescribing certain drugs to relieve the headache. For example, propranolol would not be prescribed for a patient with asthma. Neurologic deficits should be noted.
—A CAT scan may be done on selected patients.
—Skull films may be done.
—EEG is infrequently used.
—Lumbar puncture may be done if the patient demonstrates signs of meningeal irritation, such as a stiff neck and fever along with the headache.
—Cerebral angiography may be rarely used, and then only if the patient has a persistent neurologic deficit along with the headache.

A. Low Back Pain

1. General Information
—It is difficult to quantify the suffering with low back pain. The patient may not appear to be in pain.

—It has been estimated that 93 million workdays are lost in the United States each year due to back problems.

—Americans spend $5 billion each year for tests and therapies for relief of low back pain.

—At least 8 million people in the United States have a back impairment, of which approximately 500,000 are due to work-related injuries.

—Acute low back pain is almost always caused by a traumatic event.

—Chronic low back pain may have a less clear cause.

—The most common cause of low back pain is lumbosacral disc disease. If pain radiates into the leg, the usual cause is a herniated disc. Ninety-five percent of involved discs are between L4–5 or L5–S1 vertebral bodies. The two main elements in the pathology of a disc degeneration problem are degenerative changes in the disc itself and secondary damage to adjacent neural tissue.

—Causes of low back pain may include inflammation, structural disorders, neoplastic disease, metabolic disturbance, referred pain, and nonspecific back pain.

—It is commonly believed by many that there is a relationship between emotional stress and back pain. That does not rule out the possibility of serious pathology in a patient who presents with nonspecific back pain, however.

1. Medical Management

—Surgery may be performed on herniated or extruded intervertebral discs to relieve pressure on spinal nerves. The surgery, however, cannot completely reverse the effects of neural injury. So far, surgery has not solved the problem of chronic neural injury and the accompanying chronic pain. Surgery may consist of laminectomy or fusion.

—Conservative therapy includes bedrest, analgesics, muscle relaxants, instructions about body mechanics, heat or cold application, massage, and physical therapy. Some physicians recommend heat application for only about 30 minutes every 2 hours. Otherwise, there may be a lactic acid buildup in the painful area.

—Antibiotics may be used in cases of infection.

—A brace or corset may be useful in a patient with poor musculature or an elderly person with spondylosis who cannot tolerate an exercise regime. In general, however, there is less use of immobilizing devices today than several years ago. Immobilization is thought to cause soft tissue contracture and muscle atrophy.

—Epidural blocks may be used in patients with inflammation around nerve roots, as well as antiinflammatory medications.

—Traction may be used, although it currently appears that it may be that enforced bedrest rather than the actual traction is most helpful in relief of the low back pain.

—Biofeedback and hypnosis may be an aid in relieving or coping with chronic low back pain.

—Transcutaneous electrical nerve stimulation (TENS) involves implantation of stimulating devices around peripheral nerves to block pain sensations. It decreases pain perception.

—Deep brain stimulation (DBS) is a method of modulating communication of pain information to the brain. The analgesic effect produced by DBS is a result of activation of descending inhibitory systems originating from structures in the midbrain and brainstem. These inhibiting systems modulate or inhibit pain information leaving the spinal cord. This pain management technique results in pain inhibition of a specific nociceptor effect. Areas not inhibited by stimulation are still responsive to pain stimuli. DBS and morphine analgesia share overlapping opiate receptor sites in the brain.

The procedure may involve two stages of surgical intervention. The first is done under local anesthesia with patient participation and involves insertion of leads into the target sites of the brain, with attachment to an implanted electrode. The second step in the surgical procedure involves replacing the temporary percutaneous leads with chronic extender leads (internalization). There is a subclavicular receiver with an extending cable from it that is tunneled under the skin up behind the ear and connects to the extensions of the implanted electrode. (Fig. 13.1)

—Some researchers indicate that there are placebo-responders and placebo-nonresponders. When some patients are approached with what they believe to be an active drug, the suggestion of pain relief may in itself be a

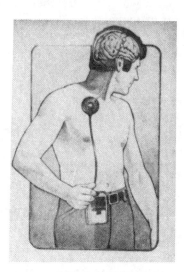

Figure 13.1. A chronic deep brain stimulation system. (Reproduced with permission from Williams A: Deep Brain Stimulation—A Contemporary Methodology for Chronic Pain. *J Neurosurg Nsg,* 16(1):5, 1984.)

stimulus for production of endorphins, which produce analgesia. A drug regimen in which an active drug is alternated with a placebo may be effective in pain relief as well as in reducing the risk of drug dependence, physiological and psychological.

—Surgical procedures such as cordotomy, rhizotomy or sympathectomy may be considered for intractable pain, as seen sometimes in cancer patients.

—Epidural or intrathecal morphine administration with an implantable infusion pump may be used, particularly in cancer patients with intractable pain. These methods of administration relieve pain without depressing the central nervous system; they provide for rapid pain relief; they provide an extended time of pain control; and generally they cause minimal side effects.

2. Diagnostic Tests

—Range of motion of joints and the effect of motion on the pain should be determined. Pain from areas such as the hip may be referred.

—Muscle spasm and tenderness to percussion and deep pressure may suggest radicular irritation.

—Rectal and vaginal examination should be performed so that local lesions and involvement of accessible lumbodorsal plexuses can possibly be ruled out.

—Straight leg raising should be performed by the patient. Pain and limited movement may be seen with radiculopathy, especially that which occurs with herniated lumbar or lumbosacral discs. Lasegue's sign refers to the pain along the sciatic nerve when it is stretched by flexing the thigh on the abdomen and the leg is extended at the knee.

—Patrick's sign should be tested for. If present, it is an indication of hip joint disease. The heel of the painful extremity is placed on the opposite knee while the patient is supine. The affected knee remains elevated and cannot be depressed toward the bed without producing pain.

—Spine x-rays may show loss of normal spinal curvature, scoliosis, and narrowing of the intervertebral disc.

—Electromyography (EMG) may be done to help localize the site of a ruptured disc.

—Lumbar puncture may be done to examine the cerebrospinal fluid. For example, elevated CSF protein may be seen with tumors of the spinal cord.

—Myelogram may be performed, especially if a tumor is suspected.

—A definitive diagnostic aid in cases of disc space infection comes from tests such as a gallium scan and total body scan.

—Preoperative evaluation may include testing psychological and/or personality factors. The Minnesota Multiphasic Personality Inventory, particularly the hypochondriasis and hysteria scales, has been a fairly acurate predictor of success of surgical intervention.

SUGGESTED READINGS

Barnett D, Hair B: Use and effectiveness of transcutaneous electrical nerve stimulation in pain management. *J Neurosurg Nsg* 13(6):323–325, 1981.

Bartorelli D: Low back pain: a team approach. *J Neurosurg Nsg* 15(1):41–44, 1983.

Dalessio D: Migraine headaches. *Hosp Med* 21(3):214–247, 1985.

Raimond J, Taylor J: *Neurological Emergencies*. Rockville, MD, Aspen Systems, 1986.

Rudy E: *Advanced Neurological and Neurosurgical Nursing*. St. Louis, CV Mosby, 1984.

Wallace K, Hays J: Nursing management of chronic pain. *J Neurosurg Nsg* 14(4):185–191, 1982.

CHAPTER **14**

Rehabilitation

Some form of rehabilitation therapy is often needed for patients with neurologic disorders. Deficits may result from head injury, spinal cord injury, degenerative disorders, or cerebrovascular disease, as discussed in the previous chapters. The deficits may be motor, cognitive, sensory, perceptual, a cranial nerve problem, or a communication problem.

There are some geeneral principles of rehabilitation regardless of the deficit. Rehabilitation involves not only a focus on helping the patient become as functionally independent as is physiologically possible; it is also intervention in helping the patient learn to live with his disability in his own environment in a way that is functional and satisfying. We may help a patient regain the skills of ADL (activities of daily living), but we must also prepare the patient to participate in adult life in the community. We need to be aware of the patient's concerns and goals, such as educational and professional goals, leisure time activities, economic security, productive employment, and role within the family.

Rehabilitation nursing involves not only restoration but prevention (especially in the neurologically impaired patient) and maintenance. Many neurologically involved patients are immobile or partially immobile. That makes skin care, pulmonary care, positioning, range of motion, maintenence of urinary and bowel continence all extremely important. If a patient develops a complication, such as a decubitus or a contracture, the whole rehabilitation program is affected and slowed down. The patient may not have the energy to fight a complication and do the activities required of a rehabilitation program. So the nurse's role is multifaceted.

Rehabilitation is also an interdisciplinary effort. The nurse, physician, physiatrist, physical therapist, occupational therapist, speech therapist, social worker, psychologist or psychiatrist, vocational counselor, recreational therapist, and dietician all have specific roles to play in the process. Other disciplines may even be brought in on a consultation basis.

Rehabilitation should begin at the time of admission for the acute event. It is a process, rather than a program beginning in a tertiary setting. The process of rehabilitation may begin as early as in the intensive care unit. A therapeutic program can be developed while the patient is at any level of recovery.

I. COGNITIVE REHABILITATION

Cognition is the basic mental structure that is the product of a series of repeated interactions between an individual and the environment. Cognition is the manner in which we organize information. After brain injury, our cognitive structure may be scrambled, causing impairment in organizing thoughts, concentrating, analyzing, sequencing, and of long- and short-term memory.

Rancho Los Amigo Rehabilitation Hospital has developed a rating scale to help assess an individual's cognitive level of functioning. The scale does not require the patient's cooperation for the assessment, because it is based on behavioral descriptions of responses to stimuli.

A. Cognitive Levels of Functioning

Level I—No response
The patient appears asleep and is completely unresponsive to any stimuli.

Level II—Generalized response
The patient's responses are limited, inconsistent, and generalized and nonpurposeful. The response may be the same to different types of stimuli, and is usually delayed. The earliest response is to deep pain.

Level III—Localized response
The patient reacts specifically to stimuli but not consistently. There may be head-turning toward a verbal stimulus, or simple withdrawal from a painful stimulus, or focusing on an object. There may be following of simple verbal commands, although usually delayed. The patient may show some awareness of himself and discomfort in his environment, demonstrated by pulling at his catheter or nasogastric tube or pulling against restraints.

Level IV—Confused, agitated response
This is a hyperactive state in which the patient's response is mostly to his internal confusion. The patient's behavior is nonpurposeful relative to the immediate environment and verbalization is inappropriate or incoherent. The patient may confabulate, have a lack of short-term recall, and may react to past events rather than the current environment. Hostility and combativeness may be shown. There is only gross attention to the environment and it is very brief, and selective attention is often nonexistent.

Level V—Confused inappropriate response
There may be agitation at this level, but it is usually a result of external stimuli, and it is often out of proportion to the stimuli. The patient follows simple commands fairly consistently, but for complex commands needs structure and frequent redirection. He is highly distractable. Memory is impaired. Verbalization may be inappropriate, confusing the past and present, but social-automatic verbalization may be carried on briefly. There is a lack of initiation of functional tasks. He is unable to learn new information. The patient may wander if not supervised.

Level VI—Confused, appropriate response
At this level, the patient is functional for activities of daily living, and has increased awareness of self, family, and basic needs. He does not wander. He follows simple directions consistently and demonstrates carry-over for activities he has learned. Long-term memory is better than short-term. He realizes he does not know certain things. Goal-directed behavior can be performed with outside direction. Information still cannot be processed well enough for the patient to predict or anticipate events. He is inconsistently oriented to time and place. Some recognition of some staff may be evident.

Level VII—Automatic, appropriate response
The patient appears appropriate and does daily routines automatically with minimal confusion but recall of what he has been doing is imparied. There is increased awareness of the environment. He initiates tasks or social and recreational activities. Judgment remains imparied. There is a lack of insight into his condition. Problem solving is very difficult. Carry-over for new learning is accomplished at a decreased rate. Minimal supervision for his safety is needed.

Level VIII—Purposeful, appropriate response
At this level, the patient is functional within society, but his social, intellectual, and emotional capacities may not be back to the baseline level prior to injury. He is alert, oriented, able to recall and integrate past and recent events. There is carry-over for new learning if it is acceptable to him and to his life role. He needs no supervision once tasks are learned. The quality and rate of processing information and abstract reasoning is still impaired. Tolerance for, and judgment in, emergency or unusual circumstances is poor.

B. Cognitive Management

Most recovery of cognitive function occurs during the first six months after injury. The recovery potential diminishes after that period. Generally, patients at Levels I, II, and III need stimulation, those at Levels IV, V, and VI need structure, and those at Levels VII and VIII need a community approach.

1. Levels I, II, III
Goals: to provide sensory input and elicit responses with increased quality, frequency, rate, duration, and variety.

—The patient has the capacity to generate responses to certain stimuli. The type of stimuli best responded to, the time of day the patient is most alert, and the variety of responses elicited should all be assessed and used for maximal results.
—Stimulation sessions should be brief but frequent.
—The presentation of stimuli should be in an organized manner, focusing on one sensory input channel at a time.

Visual stimulation

- Provide familiar objects and pictures within the patient's visual field.
- Provide visual orientation by having the patient sit in a chair or stand on a tilt table.
- Intermittent use of television will provide visual and auditory stimulation as long as it is not left on for long periods, as it then becomes "white noise" and attention to it diminishes.
- Use familiar objects, family pictures, or bright objects to have the patient focus on and track from one periphery of vision to the other.
- Provide a nondistracting environment while presenting the organized stimuli.

Auditory stimulation

- Staff and family should be encouraged to talk to the patient. Staff should explain to the patient who they are and what they are going to do.
- Family members can make tape recordings that may be played for the patient.
- Intermittent use of radio and television is helpful.
- Loud noises may be used for stimulation. If the patient response is posturing, this should not be used.

Olfactory stimulation

- The olfactory nerve is the most frequently injured cranial nerve in head injury, so stimulation of olfaction may not be productive.
- A variety of odors, such as the patient's favorite perfume or shaving lotion, may be held under the nose to see if the patient responds.
- If the patient has a tracheostomy, air is not exchanged through the nostrils, so this is ineffective. Presence of a feeding tube in one nostril reduces the sense of smell.

Cutaneous stimulation

- Staff and family should be encouraged to touch the patient.
- Response to noxious stimulation is often first to return, so pin prick or pinching may be tried.
- A variety of textures should be used with which to touch or rub the patient's skin.
- Bathing the patient provides total body cutaneous stimulation. The pressure with which the washcloth is used can be varied.
- Different temperatures can be introduced to the patient by rubbing an extremity with an ice bag or a hot water bottle.

Kinesthetic stimulation

- Turning the patient in bed or ranging his extremities or getting him up in a chair or on a tilt table or rolling him on a ball all provide the patient with an awareness of his body in space.

- Protective or balance reactions should be observed for. Place the patient in an uncomfortable position to see if he tries to move out of it.

Oral stimulation

- Routine oral hygiene gives stimulation, as does using flavored agents such as lemon swabs.
- Various tastes may be placed on the tongue.
- Perioral stimulation can be done with ice cubes, cotton swabs, etc.
- Level III patients may begin oral feeding if they have control to position the food for swallowing and have a swallow and cough reflex.

Vestibular stimulation

- A rocking bed or board may be used at different speeds of movement.

2. Level IV

Goal: to decrease agitation and increase awareness of the environment.

- —The stimuli that exacerbate the agitation and those that minimize it should be determined, if possible.
- —This phase of recovery generally persists for 2 to 4 weeks.
- —No functional goals can be set during this level, because the patient is responding primarily to his internal confusion and he is not cooperative with a structured plan of intervention.
- —Remove as many devices that may contribute to the agitation, such as nasogastric tubes, intravenous lines, and restraints as possible.
- —Avoid leaving the patient alone, unless human contact seems to make the agitation worse. When no one can be in the room, a tape recording of familiar voices can be played.
- —Provide a quiet environment without a lot of activity.
- —Explain to the patient who you are and what you plan to do. Frequent orientation is necessary.
- —Use a calm voice and manner around the patient. If the staff becomes angry or irritable with the patient, his agitation will increase. Touch may help to calm him.
- —Place no demands on the patient to follow through with tasks. He may participate in ball-throwing or other gross motor activities. He may do automatic tasks of self-care.
- —Take care if the patient is combative to prevent injury to the patient and to staff.
- —Psychotropic drugs should be avoided if possible. They may add to the agitation by increasing the internal confusion and lengthen the recovery time.

3. Levels V and VI

Goals: to decrease confusion and incorporate improved cognitive abilities into functional activity.

—Structure will provide organization of the external environment for the patient, since he is unable to do it for himself.
—During these stages, therapy includes reestablishing the patient's cognitive structures in a hierarchal sequence:
  • Attention,
  • Selective attention,
  • Analysis,
  • Discrimination,
  • Immediate and recent memory,
  • Sequencing,
  • Organization,
  • Association and categorization,
  • Integration.
  Work on one of these sequences is started with a reduced amount, reduced complexity, and reduced duration that is gradually increased, according to the patient's cognitive capacity.
—Consistency and predictability must be maintained.
  • Define expectations.
  • Keep the confused patient's environment constant.
  • Provide memory aids within visual range of the patient (for example, calendar, clock, daily schedule).
  • Minimize environmental distractions.
  • The nursing and therapy personnel should be the same daily. Relief staff should be the same to minimize number of new people with whom the patient must interact.
  • Each interaction with the patient should begin with introduction, orientation, and the purpose of interaction.
—High Level V and Level VI patients may be grouped with higher level patients for peer modeling of appropriate behaviors and orientation to reality. This may be done through joint activities.
—A list of daily activities should be typed and numbered in the sequence in which they should be done throughout the day (for example, a list for morning ADL, a list for preparing for bed at night).
—Structure may be reduced as the patient's cognitive capacity increases.
—Familiar games learned prior to injury may help to increase attention, memory, and appropriate social interaction.

4. Levels VII and VIII

Goals: to integrate increased cognitive function, with minimal structuring, into functional community activities.

—Activities that integrate cognitive growth into demands of the community are divided into three phases:
- Activities related to self,
- Activities related to home,
- Activities related to the community.

As the patient moves from one phase to the next, the demands become progressively increased as the structure and assistance are decreased. Rehearsal of activities may be done in the hospital prior to discharge.

—Typically, at the time of hospital discharge both the patient and family perceive the patient's level of functional potential to be above what it actually is.

—Prior to discharge there should be a reduction of structure in the physical environment.
- Number of staff interacting with the patient may be increased.
- Patient and staff may evaluate the use of time.
- Staff must accept patient noncompliance with parts of the program, such as being late for meetings or missed meals.

C. Psychological Aspects of Head Injury

The chart in Figure 14.1, "Psychological Stages of Recovery and Adjustment," demonstrates chronological manifestations of psychological adjustment of a patient through the rehabilitation process. The phases of recovery are impact, retreat, acknowledgment or avoidance, and adaptation. It is helpful to identify behaviors at these stages so the rehabilitative intervention can be appropriate and therapeutic.

It is really the family who feels the impact phase. The patient often does not remember the accident or the time immediately following it.

Primary variables are usually organically based, resulting from the insult. They occur at lower cognitive levels (I–V). As the patient's cognitive level increases, the primary characteristics tend to resolve, as other psychological variables (secondary personality traits) appear. Secondary characteristics are normal feelings about what has happened to the patient. These traits are pathological only in the context of what the patient does about these feelings. For example, does he deal with what has happened directly or does he deny these feelings?

The retreat behaviors are ways the patient may deal with the secondary feelings. Acknowledgement traits resemble secondary or feeling types of responses. Retreat-avoidance resembles defensive behaviors.

The patient's preinjury level of psychological functioning is very significant in terms of prognosis. If a patient has already dealt with stressful situations with retreat-avoidance or pathological behaviors prior to injury, our intervention will not likely change the same behaviors demonstrated postinjury.

Psychological intervention is usually most effective at the acknowledge-

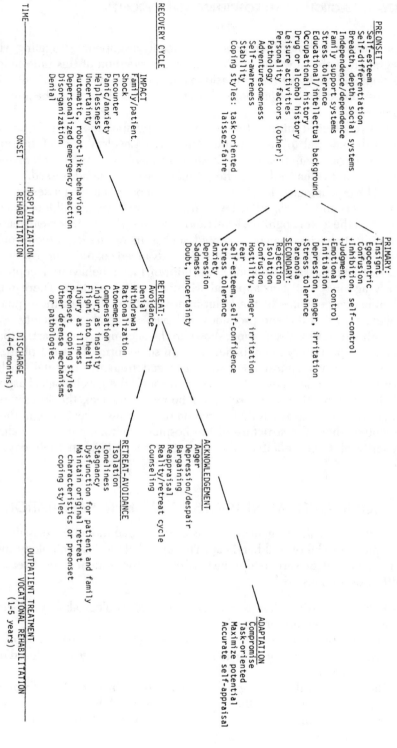

Figure 14.1. Psychological Stages of Recovery and Adjustment (Reproduced with permission from Rancho Los Amigos Hospital, Inc. *Rehabilitation of the Head Injured Adult.* 1980, p. 57.)

ment phase, during which patient and family are openly struggling with integration of the new and old identities. Intervention at this time helps the patient and family with the transition and adjustment. If the patient is in the retreat phase, he is often more resistant to outside help with the adjustment process.

Psychological intervention in cognitive rehabilitation usually progresses from the general to the specific. Patients at Levels V and VI and upward usually begin group treatment. Closer to discharge, the intervention needs to be more individualized. Specific problems need to be addressed.

The psychological levels through which a patient often passes on the way to recovery and the cognitive levels are similar to levels of childhood development. At the lower cognitive levels and at some early psychological phases, for example, behaviors may be accepted, such as incontinence, which would not be accepted if the patient were at a more advanced cognitive or psychological level. That is the same situation with children, that is, behaviors accepted at an early age may not gain approval when the child is older. There must be therapeutic guidance of the brain-injured patient through these phases of recovery so that the end product is behavior acceptable to society.

An interesting observation, shown in the accompanying chart, is that 4 to 6 months postinjury many patients are in some form of retreat phase. This, however, is when most are also discharged from the hospital. So before patients have really been able to work through the psychological aspects of their situation, they are discharged home. Many lack the insight due to cognitive deficit to assess their situation realistically. Often, once in the community without the structure of the hospital environment, they realize the severity of their deficit or the impact of the injury on their day-to-day functioning.

II. SOME ASSESSMENT TOOLS TO AID IN REHABILITATION

The World Health Organization has a conceptual model for classifying impairment, disability, and handicap. This model clarifies terminology and aids in assessment of various dimensions of the consequences of disease. The WHO definitions are:

—Impairment is any loss or abnormality of psychological, physiological, or anatomic structure or function.
—Disability is any restriction or lack (resulting from an impairment) of ability to perform an activity in the manner or within the range considered normal for a human being.
—Handicap is a disadvantage for a given individual, resulting from an impairment or disability, that limits or prevents fulfillment of a role normal (depending on age, sex, and social and cultural factors) for that individual.

So an impairment is the primary deficit, while a disability represents functional limitations, usually assessed by rehabilitation staff. Handicap refers to a social disadvantage.

Until recently, there were no assessment tools following this model. The Minimal Record of Disability has been used for assessing patients with multiple sclerosis. It now conforms with the WHO descriptions of impairment, disability, and handicap. It is hoped that other tools can be made compatible with the same model for other disease assessments. This would make communication among health professionals more uniform.

There are many scales with which to assess a patient's function. The MRD is specific to evaluation of MS dysfunction and is used with the Kurtzke Status Scale, so that the amount of neurological impairment is used for the overall evaluation.

Scales useful in assessing activities of daily living are the Kenny Self-Care Evaluation, the Barthel Index, and PULSES. The latter evaluated *P*hysical condition, *U*pper extremities, *L*ower extremities, *S*ensory components, *E*xcretory function, and mental and emotional *S*tatus.

Tools that assess disability may be helpful in the rehabilitation of a patient. They may demonstrate patient progress over time. Some help identify educational needs of the patient. Some may help determine a patient's eligibility for therapeutic trials involving drugs or other agents. A tool may show in measurable terms whether a disease process is active and how it is affecting the patient's daily activities. Some tools may identify patient needs for medical or psychological intervention. Outcomes of therapeutic interventions may be measured by assessment tools.

The MRD has had much initial acceptance as an international scale useful for cross-cultural comparisions, and work in underway to modify it for other conditions, such as stroke.

III. FAMILY INVOLVEMENT IN REHABILITATION

People with neurologic disease or injury have become a significant social concern. As technology to save lives improves, more and more people who would have died of their disease or injury are today being saved. Many of those saved are maintained at greatly reduced functional levels. This impacts on society, the family and, certainly, the patient.

In the case of head injury, there are factors which have been identified as helping predict outcome. These factors include age, presence of intracranial hematoma, abnormal motor responses, impaired or absent eye movements or pupillary reflexes, early hypotension, hypoxemia or hypercarbia, and presence of intracranial pressure. These predictive factors influence the patient's overall course of recovery from head injury, but it is not clear with regard to neuropsychological recovery. So attempting to give the family an indication of prognosis soon after injury may be very difficult.

Beginning in the acute stage of hospitalization, it is important to keep families well-informed and involved in as much of the care as possible. Studies have shown that relatives of critically ill patients need in descending order of importance:

—Kind, clear explanations,
—Discussion of realistic expectations,
—Emotional support,
—Financial counseling,
—Resource counseling.

Family support groups and family counselling are means of fulfilling the needs described both during the acute and rehabilitation phases. During the rehabilitation of the patient , families often describe the stress of character changes in the patient. Often, after head injury, the patient's personality is changed. This has been frequently more difficult for families to adjust to than physical disability, reduced intelligence, or financial problems. After head injury or in some disease processes, patients show decreased memory, impatience, depression, dependency, reduced ambition and initiative, temper outbursts, irritability, self-centered behavior, and inflexibility. Due to the patient's lack of insight into these behavior changes, resolution within the family is difficult. Family support groups allow ventilation and the reassuring knowledge that other families have similar problems. Methods of dealing with difficult situations may be shared. A book often recommended for families under this kind of stress is I. S. Cooper's book, *Living with Chronic Neurologic Disease*. The Rancho Los Amigos model of the psychological stages of recovery and adjustment is also helpful in understanding the long-term recovery cycle. (Fig. 14.1)

Teaching families about neurologic processes is very important. All members of the rehabilitation team have a responsibility in this area. Families should be assured that emotions such as anger, frustration, and sorrow are natural and it is all right to "complain" about the patient. Demonstration of these emotions does not mean the family is ungrateful that the patient is alive.

Families should be encouraged to take time away from the patient and do activities of interest to them. They should not change their whole life style to revolve only around the disabled or impaired individual. Outside social contacts should be maintained.

Unlike many other aspects of nursing, rehabilitation is a slow process, requiring unusal patience and dedication. A comprehensive approach is necessary and this certainly must include the family and caregiver. The long-term reward of this comprehensive rehabilitation intervention with a patient with neurologic impairment is the knowledge that a person has been helped to achieve maximal potential.

SUGGESTED READINGS

Cooper IS: *Living with Chronic Neurologic Disease.* New York, WW Norton, 1976.

Habermann B: Cognitive dysfunction and social rehabilitation in the severely head-injured patient. *J Neurosurg Nsg* 14(5):220–224, 1982.

Holland N, Francabandera F, Wiesel-Levison P: International scale for assessment of disability in multiple sclerosis. *J Neurosci Nsg* 18(1):39–44, 1986.

Mauss-Clum N, Ryan M: Brain injury and the family. *J Neurosurg Nsg* 13(4):165–169, 1981.

Rancho Los Amigos Hospital, Inc., *Rehabilitation of the Head Injured Adult,* 1980.

SECTION 2

NEUROSCIENCE NURSING

15

Health Perception-Health Management Pattern

The health perception-health management pattern focuses on the patient's perceptions of health and well-being. How the patient views his health and the behaviors required to maintain health provide the nurse with substantial clues as to the patient's ability to care for himself. Some patients with neurologic impairments will be cared for in a hospital while others will be cared for at home. The nurse must ensure that the patient and family know and understand the care required.

The nursing diagnosis that is most useful for patients with neurologic injury or dysfunction is potential for injury.

POTENTIAL FOR INJURY

Patients with neurologic injury or dysfunction are at risk for injury for many reasons. They may be immunosuppressed, have a cognitive disruption that leaves them with poor judgment in safety matters, or they may have a motor-sensory impairment putting them at risk for falls. An altered level of consciousness potentiates the risk of complications such as skin breakdown, loss of muscle and joint functions, and development of peripheral thrombosis.

NURSING DIAGNOSIS

Potential for injury—trauma related to:

—Altered thought processes.
—Impaired self-protective mechanism.
—Immobility
—Neuromuscular deficit.

—Side effects of medications.
—Environmental hazards.
—Seizure activity.
—Disorientation.
—Sensory-perceptual alteration: visual, kinesthetic.
—Impaired self-protective mechanisms.
—Neurologic deficits.
—Environmental hazards.
—Decreased level of responsiveness.

GOALS

The patient and family will be aware of safety factors and potential complications with regard to the patient's specific deficit; the patient will be free from physical injury; family members will know what steps to take when the patient has a seizure.

INTERVENTIONS

—Teach the family to assess the home environment for hazards (for example, throw rugs, stairs without railings, clutter); recommend environmental changes to ensure the highest level of safety (for example, grab bar in the bathroom, elevated toilet seat).
—Do not allow unsteady patients to walk unassisted.
—Review side effects of medications; be alert for potential problems.
—Teach family to recognize side effects and to report them.
—Ensure that disoriented patients do not roam unattended; encourage patient to wear identification bracelet.
—Encourage correct use of assistive devices for patients who are weak; evaluate safe use.
—Teach self-protective actions (for example, if visual field is impaired, teach patient to move head in order to scan a room; if patient has right-sided weakness, teach to approach stairs so that railing can be held with left hand).
—Recommend referral to home health agency for additional follow up and support; ensure that someone is available to assist patient upon return home.
—Encourage family members to take time out from their daily routine in order to do something for themselves.
—Pad bedrails for hospitalized patients with unpredictable seizures; keep bed in low position at all times, side rails up, padded tongue blade and oral airway at bedside with suction available.
—Administer medications (for example, anticonvulstants, steriods) on time;

SEIZURE ACTIVITY SHEET

Patient's Name ______________________________

Room No. ______________________ Age ________

Physician ______________________________

Date	Time	Before		During						Other	After				Nurse's Initials
		Warning Signs	Part of Body Where Seizure Began	General or Localized	Type of Movement	Duration of each Phase: Tonic	Duration of each Phase: Clonic	Level of Consciousness	Pupils		Behavior	Paralysis	Location of Paralysis	Sleep	

Figure 15.1. Seizure activity chart. (Reproduced with permission from Hickey J: *The Clinical Practice of Neurological and Neurosurgical Nursing.* Philadelphia, JB Lippincott, 1981.

monitor effectiveness; stress to the patient and family the importance of taking medications as ordered.

—Determine level of consciousness and behavior every 2–4 hours since seizures may be manifested by changes in behavior, such as staring into space.

—Observe patient experiencing seizures for onset (beginning of seizure, aura, epileptic cry); duration (onset to completion); motor activity (parts of the body involved, symetrical or unilateral movement); level of consciousness; incontinence.

—Use flow sheet to document information (see Figure 6.1).

—Remove environmental hazards (chairs, loosen restrictive clothing).

—Maintain patient's airway with oral airway or bite block; DO NOT insert airway or bite block if teeth are clenched.

—Protect patient's head (place a pillow or lap between patient's head and the floor).

—Do not restrain limbs; rather protect them from injury.

—Turn to side once seizure is completed to prevent aspiration of secretions; reorient as needed; observe for weakness or paralysis.

—Provide calm, quiet environment for patient to sleep after siezure; conduct a postictal assessment to determine possible injuries.

—Monitor for changes in appearance of urine (red or cola colored urine may be an indication of rhabdomyolysis or myoglobinuria).

—Teach family to protect patient from injury during seizure.

—Ensure that family and friends know to follow previously listed safety measures.

—Refer to Epilepsy Foundation of America for information; provide a list of patient family support and education groups.

—Encourage participation in the Med-Alert program.

EVALUATION CRITERIA

The patient and family

—Remove all environmental hazards.
—Use assistive devises.
—List resources available.

The patient

—Is free from seizure-activity injury.
—Calls for assistance as needed.

The family

—Knows appropriate action to take should a seizure occur.

CHAPTER **16**

Nutritional-
Metabolic Pattern

The nutritional-metabolic functional health pattern guides the nurse in the assessment of metabolic balance. The nurse focuses on the food and fluid intake of the patient, including but not limited to type, quantity, pattern, and the effect on the body systems. Imbalances are most readily identified by changes in blood chemistry, body temperature and weight, and the condition of the skin, hair, nails, and teeth. Patients experiencing neurologic impairments require increased energy to heal, yet may be limited in the manner in which they take in food.

The nursing diagnoses that are most useful for patients experiencing neurologic injury or dysfunction and associated with the functional nutritional-metabolic health pattern include excess in fluid volume, nutrition lower than body requirements, alteration in oral mucous membranes, fluid volume deficit, impaired skin integrity, ineffective thermoregulation, and potential for infection.

Excess in Fluid Volume. Excess fluid volume may be a side effect of steroid therapy, concomitant injuries, or disease processes in the neurologic population.

Nutritional Deficit. Patients with neurologic dysfunction have many reasons for potentially altered nutritional status. These include nerve damage, resulting in muscular dysfunction or paralysis, and altered level of consciousness, which may preclude obtaining adequate nutrition. Inadequate nutrition may also be iatrogenic (for example, an imposed fluid restriction or NPO status). There may be increased energy expenditure after neurologic injury, and nurses need to ensure the nutritional needs are met, regardless of the patient's condition.

Alteration in Oral Mucous Membranes. A patient with neurologic involvement may develop an alteration in the oral mucous membrane due to several factors. Head injured patients are frequently placed on a fluid restriction or are NPO for several days. Ineffective oral hygiene may be an issue, especially during the time a patient is orally intubated. Additionally, mouth breathing and some medications may dry out the oral mucosa. Patients with neurologic problems may not be physically able to perform oral hygiene, or they may not be cognitively aware that they should do it.

Fluid Volume Deficit. Patients experiencing neurologic illness or injury may not be able to take in adequate amounts of fluid to meet physiologic needs. Factors that may contribute to the fluid deficit include immobility, confusion, weakness, and total dependence.

Impaired Skin Integrity. Patients with neurologic injury or disease frequently suffer from impaired skin integrity due to altered reflexes and sympathetic tone, loss of sensation from certain body parts, altered nutrition, and immobility due to an altered level of consciousness. Disturbance in skin integrity is most often preventable.

Ineffective Thermoregulation. Patients experiencing a disruption of sympathetic pathways between the hypothalamus and the peripheral blood vessels (e.g., with a spinal cord injury), may have difficulty with thermoregulation as evidenced by labile temperatures.

Potential for Infection. Patients with neurologic diagnoses and those being treated for neurologic disorders are at risk for infection by the very nature of the diagnosis or as a possible side effect of the treatment. Surgery interrupts the skin integrity, as do numerous catheters and other invasive procedures that may be needed. Immobility or bedrest places a patient at risk for pulmonary complications. The NPO status may deplete the nutritional state. Steriods may cause immunosuppression and make a patient more susceptible to a nosocomial infection.

NURSING DIAGNOSIS

Alteration in fluid volume: excess related to

—Neuro/hormonal dysfunction,
—Side effects of drugs.

Fluid volume deficit related to

—Neuro/hormonal dysfunction,
—Side effects of drugs.

GOALS

The patient will regain and maintain adequate hydration; will have a balanced fluid intake and output.

INTERVENTIONS

—Monitor vital signs and hemodynamic parameters at least every 4 hours.
—Monitor for signs of *fluid overload* (for example, dyspnea or tachypnea,

dysrhythmias, gallop rhythm, distention of neck veins, edema, increased abdominal girth).

—Monitor for signs of *fluid deficit* (for example, decreased blood pressure, urine output; poor skin turgor; dry mucous membranes; complaints of thirst).

—Monitor level of consciousness, watching for signs of increased ICP and signs of seizure activity.

—Monitor lung sounds and respirations, vital signs, and skin integrity.

—Record intake and output accurately; calculate fluid balance.

—Measure urine specific gravity every 4–8 hours.

—Weigh daily.

—Monitor electrolytes, serum albumin and hematocrit.

—Ensure accurate I.V. rate; use infusion pump whenever possible.

—Elevate head of the bed as necessary to facilitate breathing.

—Restrict or encourage fluids as indicated.

EVALUATION CRITERIA

The patient

—Has lab values within normal limits.

—Maintains clear breath sounds.

—Maintains hourly urine output between 60 ml and 120 ml.

—Has elastic skin, no edema.

NURSING DIAGNOSIS

Alteration in nutrition: less than body requirements related to

—Altered level of consciousness.

—Oral intake restrictions.

—Gastrointestinal dysfunction: nausea, vomiting, diarrhea, decreased peristalsis.

—Dysphagia, difficulty chewing.

—Pain.

—Limited ability to feed self.

—Fear of aspiration.

—Increased caloric requirements and energy expenditure.

—Cognitive impairments.

GOALS

The patient will take in sufficient nutrition to meet health needs; will maintain optimal nutritional status and fluid intake.

INTERVENTIONS

—Monitor for presence of bowel sounds; encourage feedings as soon as possible; encourage use of hyperalimentation by the physician for patients with absent bowel sounds or if feedings are not tolerated.

—Assess swallowing status, fluid intake, gag reflex, and motor skills before attempting oral feedings.

—Determine patient's caloric need and intake; collaborate with physician and dietician to assure adequate nutrition.

—Administer hyperalimentation as ordered per i.v. pump and controller to assure a constant rate of administration; monitor serum glucose if total parenteral nutrition is given.

—Administer tube feedings if patient is unable to swallow, either through nasogastric tube or gastrostomy tube; there is less chance for regurgitation around a small, weighted tube, rather than a large gastric tube, and it is less uncomfortable for the patient.

—Color tube feeding with blue food coloring if an artificial airway such as a tracheostomy is present; if the secretions suctioned are blue-tinged, the patient is probably aspirating.

—Position patient upright when eating or receiving tube feedings.

—Check gastric residuals if receiving tube feedings; feedings may be held for at least an hour if the residual is greater than 100–125 ml.

—Watch for signs of aspiration.

—Maintain patency of feeding tubes by flushing periodically with warm water.

—Provide colorful types of food in a pleasant environment.

—Assure that patient has glasses on and dentures in place when eating a meal.

—Provide an area with minimal distraction if patient is prone to aspiration, so he can pay attention to the task of eating.

—Provide environment conducive to eating (for example, removing bedpans, soiled linen, and clutter from the area).

—Determine patient's food likes and dislikes and incorporate into menu planning; encourage family to bring in favorite foods from home.

—Provide supervision for the demented patient who may forget to eat.

—Begin oral feeding with a semisolid food such as ice cream because liquids may be difficult to swallow initially.

—Offer small frequent feedings, which may be better tolerated than three larger meals a day.

—Prevent choking by having the patient's food cut up into bite-size pieces.

—Avoid use of straws, as the patient may not be able to suck on it.

—Avoid milk products if there are many secretions.

—Monitor input and output and weight changes to ensure adequate renal function, hydration, nutrition.

—Pace activities so patient is not too tired to eat.
—Minimize GI upset by administering irritating medications with food or milk when possible.

EVALUATION CRITERIA

The patient

—Maintains preillness/injury body weight.
—Experiences progressive tissue healing.
—Is free from aspiration.
—Has normal lab values.
—Participates in menu planning.

NURSING DIAGNOSIS

Alteration in oral mucous membrane related to

—Inability to perform oral hygiene.
—Fluid restriction.
—Dehydration.
—Immunosuppression.
—Invasive procedures.
—Inadequate oral intake or oral hygiene.
—Malnutrition.
—Coma.
—Placement of tube for several days.

GOALS

The patient will regain and/or maintain moist, intact oral mucous membranes; will maintain good oral hygiene.

INTERVENTIONS

—Inspect mouth and mucosa; assess color, moisture, ulcerations, odor of oral membrane and gums.
—Provide mouth care at least every 2 hours; use particular caution for patients with open areas/incisions (for example, transphenoidal lip incision) of oral mucous membranes.
—Perform oral hygiene for patient unable to do so for self.
—Give soft nonacidic foods if mucosa not intact.
—Rinse patient's mouth with diluted hydrogen peroxide after meals if signs of thrush appear.

—Perform oral hygiene on patients who are unconscious as often as needed; turn patient on side, place tongue blade to keep mouth open; brush using a solution of hydrogen peroxide and water (1:4); rinse mouth with a bulb syringe and aspirate rinse with suction.
—Moisten mouth with cracked ice; pat mouth dry and apply lip lubricant.
—Swab the mouth with diluted glycerine; brush tongue and inner cheek gently.
—Instruct patients on side effects of drugs such as phenytoin, which may cause gum hyperplasia, and about the importance of good oral hygiene.
—Evaluate patient's ability to perform oral hygiene; teach proper method of brushing teeth, flossing and cleaning dentures; encourage oral hygiene after meals and at bedtime.

EVALUATION CRITERIA

The patient

—Is free from bleeding from oral mucosa.
—Is free from thrush.

The patient or family

—Brushes and flosses patient's teeth at least 2 times a day.

NURSING DIAGNOSIS

Impaired skin integrity related to

—Immobility.
—Lack of sensation.
—Altered nutritional status.
—Hypothermia therapy.
—Trauma: invasive procedures/surgical incision.
—Bowel and/or bladder incontinence.

GOALS

The patient will maintain warm, dry, intact skin; the patient and family will perform activities to prevent skin breakdown.

INTERVENTIONS

—Observe for signs of skin irritation or redness.
—Establish a turning schedule.
—Turn and reposition patient every 2 hours if patient is unable to turn or if level of consciousness is depressed.

—Use mild soap and lotions without alcohol; alcohol has a drying effect that increases the risk of skin breakdown; massage area over bony prominences.
—Monitor temperature of bath water and any heating devices to prevent burns.
—Provide kinetic bed, flotation system, air mattress, or sheepskin to reduce pressure on bony prominences and enhance circulation.
—Keep skin dry and clean, free from urine and feces.
—Use external catheter, properly applied, on incontinent males if appropriate to keep skin free from urine.
—Use sterile technique with invasive procedures such as inserting i.v. lines or bladder catheters.
—Monitor nutrition and hydration status that may contribute to skin breakdown (for example, inadequate protein, calories, or fluid intake).
—Use measures to improve peripheral circulation (for example, range of motion exercises, thigh-high elastic stockings, pneumatic stockings) in patients who are immobile or in spinal shock.
—Instruct patient to shift weight and to evaluate skin by using a mirror to see when redness appears; tell to increase the time in any one position (up to 2 hours) as skin tolerance increases.
—Prevent overlapping skin surfaces from touching by using properly positioned pads and pillows, joint protectors; teach family how to pad bony prominences.
—Use paper or transparent tape instead of adhesive on the skin.
—Give injections in muscle with tone for better absortion and less risk of sterile abscess formation; do not administer an injection of greater than 1 ml into muscle without tone, as in a quadriplegic.
—Instruct patient to stay out of the sun if receiving radiation.

EVALUATION CRITERIA

The patient

—Is free from signs and symptoms of skin breakdown.
—Recognizes early signs and symptoms of skin breakdown.

The family

—Verbalizes understanding of and practices methods to prevent skin breakdown.

NURSING DIAGNOSIS

Ineffective thermoregulation related to

—Disruption of autonomic nervous system function.
—Coma or increased intracranial pressure.

—Head trauma or brain tumor.
—Cerebrovascular disease.
—Altered metabolic rate.

GOALS

The patient will be comfortable; will maintain normal body temperature.

INTERVENTIONS

—Control environmental temperature to patient's comfort.
—Monitor patient's vital signs and temperature at least every 4 hours.
—Observe for signs of fever (for example, hot dry skin, flushed face, malaise, rash, respiratory distress).
—Remember that administration of steroids may mask a fever.
—Use blankets, heating pads as necessary.
—Administer antipyretics as ordered; monitor effectiveness.
—Use hypo/hyperthermia blankets to cool or warm patient within normal limits.
—Provide careful skin care when on hypo/hyperthermia blanket; assess for turgor, temperature, appearance and quality of peripheral pulses.
—Consider insensible water loss from fever, which may affect total hydration when measuring intake and output.
—Observe for signs of dehydration (for example, parched mouth, furrowed tongue, dry lips).
—Increase caloric intake because of increased metabolic rate when fever is present.

EVALUATION CRITERIA

The patient

—Maintains body temperature between 36°C (96.8°F) and 37.6°C (99.7°F).

NURSING DIAGNOSIS

Potential for infection related to

—Immunosuppression.
—Altered respiratory functioning.
—Compromised nutritional status.
—Drug therapy (for example, steroids, barbiturates).
—Immobility, bedrest.
—Impaired skin integrity.

—Compromised cranial integrity (injury, surgery, ICP monitoring device).
—Invasive lines, catheters.

GOALS

The patient will be free from infection.

INTERVENTIONS

—Maintain optimal aseptic environment during bedside insertion of invasive lines; maintain a sterile occlusive dressing over catheter insertion sites.
—Check i.v. sites every shift for signs of infection (for example, erythema, drainage, tenderness, induration) and change if necessary; follow hospital protocol for changing tubing on i.v. lines.
—Change all dressing at least daily so the wound is seen.
—Monitor temperature, vital signs at least every 4 hours for indication of infection.
—Monitor urine glucose; glycosuria and hyperglycemia may be early signs of possible catheter-related sepsis.
—Monitor white blood cell count.
—Instruct patient and family in ways to prevent infection.
—Wash hands between caring for one patient and another to prevent possible cross-contamination.
—Follow isolation techniques if the patient has an infection.
—Change ventilator and oxygen tubing per protocol.
—Monitor visitors for respiratory infections and discourage their presence if infectious.
—Be aware of side effects of drugs given.
—Protect immunologically compromised persons, such as patients with AIDS or on steroids from nosocomial secondary infections.
—Maintain skin integrity by keeping patient clean and dry and changing positions if patient is unable to do so for self; use air mattress or sheepskin as indicated.
—Assess otorrhea or rhinorrhea for presence of CSF, which puts the patient at risk for meningitis.
—Do not pack ear or nose if CSF leak suspected; rather, provide a sterile field to collect drainage and notify physician.
—Watch for complications of meningitis after ventriculostomy or shunt placement (for example, nuchal rigidity, photophobia, irritation, altered LOC, headache).
—Educate patient with a shunt about early signs of shunt infection (for example, fever).

EVALUATION CRITERIA

The patient

—Demonstrates preventative methods for avoiding infection.
—Has normal WBC.
—Is afebrile.

CHAPTER 17

Elimination Pattern

Although elimination problems are rarely viewed as priorities, balance and stability is critical for health and well-being. The functional health pattern, elimination, focuses on normal elimination patterns (bowel, bladder, skin); regularity; routines; modes, quality, and quanity of excretion; and finally, changes. Patients experiencing neurologic impairment and immobility frequently have problems in these areas. Nurses and patients must focus on and solve elimination problems.

The nursing diagnoses that are most useful for patients experiencing neurologic injury or dysfunction and associated with the functional health pattern of elimination include alteration in bowel elimination (constipation, diarrhea, and incontinence) and alteration in patterns of urinary elimination.

Alteration in Bowel Elimination: Constipation, Diarrhea, Incontinence. There may be an alteration in bowel elimination from cognitive impairment, muscle weakness, or nerve impairment. Altered diet, fluid restriction, effects of anesthesia, immobility, interruption of usual bowel routine, tube feeding intolerance, lack of privacy in the hospital, pain medications, spinal nerve compression, paralytic ileus, impaired communication, failure to respond to cues, or absence of sensation or volitional control may all contribute to an altered bowel pattern.

Alteration in Patterns of Urinary Elimination. Neuromuscular impairment and loss of sensation and mobility may cause bladder dysfunction. Upper motor neuron injuries leave the micturition center intact, so reflex activity of the bladder is preserved. Lower motor neuron injuries destroy the reflex activity for micturition, and the bladder is flaccid. The detrusor muscle, however, has some inherent contractile ability that is useful in bladder emptying. There is a high social value placed on continence, so patients with altered patterns of urinary elimination should be helped with a bladder retraining program suitable to their level of injury and impairment.

NURSING DIAGNOSIS

Alteration in bowel elimination: constipation, incontinence related to
—Immobility, decreased physical activity.

—Depressed level of consciousness.
—Spinal nerve sompression.
—Absence of sensation and/or volitional control.
—Decreased peristalsis.
—Inability to communicate needs.
—Weakness.

GOALS

The patient will eliminate soft-formed stools at regular intervals.

INTERVENTIONS

—Auscultate bowel sounds daily; they may be absent during spinal shock or may be a high tinkling if an ileus is present.
—Monitor for abdominal distention if bowel sounds are absent or diminished; loss of peristalsis (related to impaired innervation) paralyzes the bowel, causing an ileus and bowel distention; the latter may precipitate autonomic dysreflexia in spinal-cord injured patients.
—Check stools for occult blood; may be a side effect of steroid or anticoagulant administration and/or stress ulcer.
—Provide privacy when patient is defecating.
—Establish a scheduled time for bowel elimination based on the patient's routine prior to hospitalization.
—Encourage fluids (2000–2400 ml/day) unless contraindicated.
—Administer stool softeners and suppositories as ordered and indicated; monitor effectiveness.
—Be aware that laxatives may be ordered to prevent the patient from straining, especially if an aneurysm or arteriovenous malformation is present and has not been surgically repaired.
—Be aware that distention may precipitate autonomic dysreflexia in spinal-cord injured patients.
—For patient with spinal cord injury, remove feces manually until rectal reflexes return; apply a generous amount of nupercainal ointment or xylocaine jelly to the rectum to anesthetize the area.
—Maintain nasogastric tube and intravenous feedings until bowel sounds are present and paralytic ileus is resolved after spinal cord injury.
—Recognize early signs and symptoms of autonomic dysreflexia thought to be due to impaction (see Table 17.1); do not attempt to remove the impaction until symptoms subside; once symptoms have resolved, manually remove the impaction.
—Use digital stimulation after each incontinent stool to ensure bowel evacuations in patient with spinal cord injury.

Table 17.1.
Signs and Symptoms of Autonomic Dysreflexia

Severe Hypertension
Pounding Headache
Flushing of Head and Neck, Engorgement of Temporal and Neck Vessels
Nasal Congestion
Sweating above Level of Injury and Piloerection
Chills without Fever

Nursing Treatment Checklist for Autonomic Dysreflexia
1. Elevate head of bed.
2. Apply blood pressure cuff and check blood pressure every one to two minutes.
    A. If BP is above 180/90 proceed to step 5.
    B. If BP is below 180/90 proceed as follows.
3. Quickly insert bladder catheter or check bladder drainage system in place to detect possible obstruction.
    A. Check to make sure plug or clamp is not in catheter or on tubing.
    B. Check for kinks in catheter or drainage tubing.
    C. Check inlet to leg bag it make sure it is not corroded.
    D. Check to make sure leg bag is not overfull.
    E. If none of these are evident, proceed to step 4.
4. Determine if catheter is plugged by irrigating the bladder slowly with no more than 30 ml of irrigation solution. Use of more solution may increase the massive sympathetic outflow already present. If symptoms have not subsided, proceed to step 5.
5. Change the catheter and empty the bladder.
6. When you are sure the bladder is empty and if BP is:
    A. Above 180/90 call physician immediately
    B. Below 180/90 proceed as follows:
       Atropine given according to physician's order. If BP rises or fails to sub-side, call physician immediately. Ismelin, Apresoline or inhaled amyl ni-trate may then be ordered by the physician. Dibenzylene may be used for chronic dysreflexia.
7. Ideally, this procedure requires 3 people: one to check the BP, one to check the drainage system, and one to notify the physician.

If bladder overdistention does not seem to be the cause of the dysreflexia,
1. Check for bowel impaction. Do not attempt to remove it, if present. Apply nupercainal ointment or xylocaine jelly to the rectum and anal area. As the area is anesthetized, the BP should fall. After the BP is again stable, using a generous amount of anesthetizing ointment or jelly, manually remove impaction.
2. Change patient's position. Pressure areas may be the source of dysreflexia.

—Stimulate the reflex bowel (for example, stroke downward on the abdomen; apply pressure in front of, in back of, and to the side of the anus) when re-training the bowel.
—Encourage patient to respond to the elimination reflex immediately.
—Provide a high-fiber diet unless otherwise indicated; offer prune juice at bedtime or 8–10 hours before planned time for defecation.
—Refer to box on page 201 for steps in bowel training program.

EVALUATION CRITERIA

The patient

—Empties bowel intentionally at specific times.
—Passes soft, formed stools.
—Is free from abdominal distention.

NURSING DIAGNOSIS

Alteration in patterns of urinary elimination: reflux, functional, total incon-tinence related to

—Lack of sensory and motor nerve innervation to the bladder.
—Spinal nerve compression.
—Indwelling catheter.
—Immobility.
—Inability to verbalize needs.
—Loss of inhibition and social expectations.

GOALS

The patient will maintain socially acceptable pattern of urinary elimination and will be free from complications associated with ineffective bladder emptying.

INTERVENTIONS

—Palpate bladder for distention at least every 4 hours, gently and carefully as this procedure can trigger autonomic dysreflexia in spinal-cord injured patients.
—Monitor and record intake and output daily.
—Note clarity, color, and odor of urine to determine concentration, possible UTI.
—Monitor lab values (for example, BUN, creatinine, white blood count) that reflect renal adequacy and presence of infection.

Steps in a Bowel Training Program

Goal: to attain and maintain bowel continence.

1. Determine bowel habits preinjury if possible.
2. Follow established bowel program. An example of a bowel program is:
   For patients who are being fed (tube feedings or regular food):
   —Colace 100 mg orally or per nasogastric tube three times a day.
   —Dulcolax suppository every night unless the patient has had a bowel movement that day.
   —Milk of magnesia 30 ml orally or per nasogastric tube every other night or even dates unless patient has had a bowel movement that day.
   For patients who are NPO:
   —Dulcolax suppository every other night on even dates.
3. Slush enema may be given every day until peristalsis is present. This consists of giving approximately a liter tap water enema, then holding the container below the level of the bed, allowing the water to return, and repeating the procedure several times.
4. Use bowel program in conjunction with digital stimulation. Digital stimulation consists of inserting a lubricated, gloved index finger into the anal sphincter, using a rotating motion of the finger around the sphincter. The sphincter will slowly dilate as the dilatation occurs. The finger is inserted to about half its length, and the circular rotation is continued for 15–20 minutes until stool passes into the rectum and is then evacuated from the rectum.
5. Once a pattern of evacuation is established, use only digital stimulation if possible, eliminating the suppository. Use only the bowel program on individuals unable to tolerate digital stimulation.
6. Use digital stimulation after each involuntary bowel movement while the bowel pattern is being established.
7. Modify the bowel program according to individual needs as determined by stool consistency.
8. Use nupercainal ointment or xylocaine jelly to insert suppository or for digital stimulation if patient is prone to episodes of autonomic dysreflexia. The ointment or jelly may be used in the rectum and around the anal sphincter prior to insertion of the suppository or finger.
9. Maintain high fluid intake when not contraindicated, for example, in cases of fluid restriction or increased intracranial pressure.
10. Use incontinence pads rather than a bedpan when giving routine bowel care. A bedpan does not work well for these reasons: it is hard and can cause pressure areas over the coccyx; it does not allow access to the anus for digital stimulation; and it can upset the spinal alignment necessary for proper healing in spinal cord injured patients.
11. Notify physician of prolonged or severe diarrhea, impaction, rectal bleeding, or hemorrhoids.

—Do not clamp a bladder catheter; if the bladder is overfull, the urine has nowhere to go but to reflux back into the kidneys.

—Begin aseptic intermittent catheterization program as soon as possible to prevent complications associated with retention of catheters (for example, infection, atonic bladder).

—Assess methods to stimulate the reflex bladder (for example, applying cold to the abdomen, stroking the inner thigh, or pulling pubic hairs).

—Promote success of the bladder program; begin catheterization every 4 hours; if volume is greater than 500 ml, catheterization may need to be

---

Steps in an Intermittent Catheterization Protocol

Goal of intermittent catheterization: To eliminate the need for an indwelling urethral or suprapubic catheter, consequently reducing the incidence of urinary tract complications, for example, infections, periurethral abscess, epididymitis, and to establish and maintain a safe catheter-free state for patients with neurogenic bladders.

1. Limit fluid intake to 600–800 ml between catheterizations.
2. Catheterize patient every 4 hours initially. When residual urine volumes are consistently less than 400 ml/two days, decrease catheterizations to every 6 hours.
3. Record voided amounts and residuals on intake and output record.
4. Decrease number of catheterizations as voiding amounts increase or residuals decrease.
5. Catheterize patient every 8 hours when residual urine volumes are consistently less than 300 ml/2 days.
6. Catheterize patient every 12 hours when residual urine volumes are consistently less than 200 ml/2 days.
7. Catheterize patient every 24 hours when residual urine volumes are consistently less than 150 ml/2 days.
8. Catheterize postvoiding every other day for one week when residuals are consistently less than 100 ml/2 days.
9. Catheterize postvoiding to measure residual urine volume every third day for one week, then once the next week, and then once a month for three months. As long as the patient is in the hospital, catheterize postvoiding to measure residual urine volume any time urine infection is demonstrated.
10. Obtain urine culture at start of the program and every 7 days thereafter.
11. When patient begins to void between catheterizations, use an external collector to maintain continence with males. Spiral it around the penis but do not overlap it.
12. Prior to catheterization procedure, assist patient to empty bladder by Credé or Valsalva maneuvers, anal dilatation, or any other method which will trigger voiding for the particular patient. Sometimes tapping or percussing the bladder with one or two fingers will initiate voiding.
13. Notify physician of difficulty with catheterization, increased sediment or mucus in urine, hematuria, or continuous high residuals (over 500 ml).

more frequent; the goal of the program is to obtain urine volumes under 500 ml.

—Keep the patient on a fluid restriction during the program not exceeding 600–800 ml between catheterizations.

—Act quickly when a spinal cord injured patient demonstrates symptoms of autonomic dysreflexia; make sure that the catheter is not kinked or obstructed; follow hospital procedure for catheter irrigation, if necessary; take appropriate step to empty patient's bladder if distended.

—If catheter in a spinal-cord injured patient has sediment in it, irrigate it with a *maximum* of 30 ml saline; more than 30 ml may increase the massive sympathetic outflow; if irrigation does not clear catheter, remove it and insert a new one.

—If patient is on steroids, perform fractional urine testing to monitor for glucose intolerance (insulin may be administered according to a sliding scale, as ordered); hyperglycemia will increase water loss and may prevent a bladder retraining program from working.

—Help family anticipate needs of the patient, such as helping to bathroom every 2 hours to prevent accidental incontinence.

—Teach to record amount and frequency of voidings if patient is voiding on his own.

—Encourage toileting routine prior to bedtime, especially with demented patients.

—Restrict fluids after 8 PM for patients who are incontinent of urine during the night.

—Monitor temperature every 8 hours, as fever may indicate bladder infection.

EVALUATION CRITERIA

The patient

—Has clear, yellow urine.
—Empties bladder intentionally at specific times.
—Is free from incontinent episodes.

CHAPTER **18**

Activity-Exercise Pattern

The activity-exercise pattern describes activities and energy expenditures, including activities of daily living, routine activities, and recreational pursuits. Many factors influence an individual's activity pattern. Patients with neurologic impairments may experience a wide variety of disturbances that interfere with normal activities (for example, neuromuscular deficits, immobility, altered respiratory and/or cardiac function).

The nursing diagnoses that are most useful for patients experiencing neurologic injury or dysfunction and associated with the functional health pattern of activity-exercise include activity intolerance, alteration in cerebral tissue perfusion, impaired gas exchange, impaired physical mobility, ineffective airway clearance, ineffective breathing pattern, and self-care deficit in feeding, bathing and hygiene, dressing and grooming, and in toileting.

Activity Intolerance. Activity intolerance in the neurologically impaired population is common. Strength and endurance may be minimal following an acute neurologic insult. Prolonged hospitalization, immobility, bedrest, pain, and a poor nutritional status may all contribute to fatigue. Dyspnea, depression, and hemiparesis may also prevent the patient from performing normal activities. Fatigue may also be a side effect of chemotherapy. If contractures develop, impaired range of motion may result, which limits activities available to the patient. Low hemoglobin, for whatever reason, also results in activity intolerance.

Alteration in Cerebral Tissue Perfusion. Altered perfusion to brain tissue is frequently caused by increased intracranial pressure (ICP). The increased ICP may be due to several causes (cerebral edema, hypotension, hypoxia, a space-occupying lesion, or direct disruption of blood flow to an area of the brain due to a thrombus or embolus) resulting in ischemic infarcted brain tissue. Sustained elevation of the ICP may impair the degree of neurologic recovery, and should be avoided if at all possible. A great deal of nursing care has a direct effect on ICP, so nurses play a vital role in maximizing the patient's outcome.

Impaired Gas Exchange, Ineffective Airway Clearance, Ineffective Breathing Pattern. Respiratory dysfunction may result from neurologic insult. The nervous system has much control over the respiratory system. The more depressed the level of consciousness, the more the patient is at risk for pulmonary complications. Particular respiratory patterns observed clinically may be indicative of where the pathology is in the brain. There are several protective reflexes regulated by the respiratory system, some of which influence respiratory rate and depth, some of which control coughing, sneezing, and yawning. Increased intracranial pressures and disorders affecting the cerebral hemispheres or the brainstem frequently cause disturbances in respiratory reflexes and respiratory rate and rhythm that may or may not influence gas exchange.

Impaired Physical Mobility. Patients experiencing neurologic illness or injuries frequently experience motor and sensory dysfunction. Motor dysfunction may manifest as weakness or paralysis, while sensory dysfunction results in paresthesia or the inability to identify stimuli. Both problems interfere with the patient's ability to move.

Self-care Deficit. There are numerous reasons for a patient experiencing neurologic injury or dysfunction to have a self-care deficit. An altered state of consciousness, confusion, muscular weakness, or paralysis of a limb or body part, visual defects or psychological problems (for example, depression) may all contribute to an inability to care adequately for oneself. The deficit may be tempory or permanent.

NURSING DIAGNOSIS

Activity intolerance related to

—Immobility.
—Weakness.
—Paralysis.
—Poor nutrition.
—Fatigue.
—Neurologic deficits.

GOALS

The patient will increase endurance from time of injury or illness; will participate in a prescribed activity program without undue fatigue.

INTERVENTIONS

—Assess the effect of neurologic impairment on patient's ability to carry out activities of daily living.
—Initiate physical and occupational therapy for patients with motor deficits as soon as possible.
—Alternate rest and activity to prevent overexertion or excessive fatigue; assist with activity as needed.

—Plan daily activities with patient so patient can anticipate upcoming ones.
—Advise a gradual return to noncompetitive activities.
—Provide meaningful activities, taking the patient's likes and dislikes into account if possible; encourage socialization as tolerated, avoid stressful activities.
—Perform and instruct patient in range-of-motion exercises to prevent muscle atrophy and contractures.
—Use bed board, foot board to prevent contractures; use decubitus-prevention measures (for example, heel and elbow protectors, egg-crate mattress).
—Monitor vital signs during activity to prevent overexertion and stress.
—Administer analgesia prior to planned activity if movement creates pain for the patient; encourage patient to participate in activities during energy peaks following administration of medication.
—Provide for muscle rest and immobility during the phase in Guillain-Barré when the muscles are sore or tender; ranging or stretching muscles during that stage may increase demyelination.
—Provide active or passive range-of-motion exercise even during the acute phase of the illness to prevent some complications of immobility.
—Promote continuation of the use of the skills and abilities the patient has intact; encourage independence as tolerated.
—Have family or caregivers of a demented patient establish a routine schedule (for example, exercise, meals, bedtime, medication); an established routine within a structured environment gives the patient some stability and security.

EVALUATION CRITERIA

The patient

—Is free from contractures.
—Tolerates desired level of activity.
—Avoids injury.

NURSING DIAGNOSIS

Alteration in cerebral tissue perfusion related to

—Interruption in cerebral blood flow (arterial, venous).
—Increased intracranial pressure.
—Loss of intracranial compliance.
—Increase in cerebral contents (for example, brain edema, mass, CSF volume).
—Pressure on vasculature.
—Intracerebral steal.

—Hypervolemia or hypovolemia
—Changes in blood pressure.
—Hemorrhage.
—Decreased cardiac output, dysrhythmias.

GOALS

The patient will maintain cerebral perfusion of at least 50 mm Hg; will maintain intracranial pressure of less than 20 mm Hg.

INTERVENTIONS

—Monitor intracranial pressure for rises.
—Maintain venous outflow from the brain by elevating the head of the bed and properly aligning head without neck flexion or head rotation.
—Minimize environmental stimuli.
—Determine the need for external stimuli when doing neuro checks; if an ICP monitoring device is in place, it may not be necessary to give the patient painful stimulation frequently to asess motor ability. (Some researchers believe that pain causes an increase in cerebral blood flow which may increase ICP due to the additional volume in the head).
—Avoid positioning patient with hips flexed over 90 degrees, which impedes venous outflow from the head because of increase intraabdominal pressure.
—Avoid or minimize frequency and duration of nursing care to prevent elevating intrathoracic or intraabdominal pressure (for example, keep airway patent; if suctioning is necessary, hyperoxygenate and hyperventilate prior to procedure; do not suction longer than 10 seconds at a time).
—Allow ICP to drop between tasks if ICP is labile (for example, do not turn, suction, take vital signs all at one time but space them); coordinate and space activities such as x-rays and range-of-motion exercises based on ICP readings; organize nursing care to allow optimal rest periods for patient.
—Check that endotracheal tube tape or tracheostomy ties are not tight enough to impede venous return from the head.
—Recognize and intervene before a critical change in vital signs may alter cerebral perfusion.
—Maintain normothermia with acetaminophen suppositories and hypothermia blankets, as ordered.
—Monitor the physiologic responses to therapy to help prevent further neurologic deficits.
—Talk to the patient, even if unconscious, explaining what you plan to do prior to inititating care, as it is uncertain what the patient perceives.
—Do not say anything in the presence of the patient that you would not say if he were awake; hearing is one of the last senses to diminish.

—Ask family members to talk to a paitent if it proves helpful in lowering the ICP.

—Calculate cerebral perfusion pressure (CPP) if an ICP monitor and an arterial line are in place to assure adequate cerebral perfusion (CPP = mean systemic arterial pressure minus the ICP).

—Turn the conscious patient instead of having him actively turn; passive turning avoids isometric contractions and a Valsalva maneuver; keep the head in alignment with the body while turning; avoid placing patient in prone or Trendelenburg position.

—Maintain proper functioning of ICP monitoring device according to institution protocol to maintain the integrity of the invasive device (that is, closed system, positioning of transducer, recalibration, system free of air).

—Monitor electrocardigraphic changes that might alter cerebral perfusion:

- S-T segment depression or elevation.
- Prolonged Q-T or Q-U intervals.
- Q waves in the standard and precordial leads.
- U waves.
- Inverted or upright broad T waves.

—Utilize restraints only when absolutely necessary, because agitation will increase ICP and reduce cerebral perfusion.

—Watch for rebound phenomenon (that is, signs of neurologic deterioration) after osmotic diuretics are given.

—Keep family informed regarding status of patient and prognosis; allow family members to participate in patient care as appropriate.

—Allow only passive range-of-motion exercises while ICP is labile.

—Monitor neurologic status and compare with patient's baseline, using objective tool such as the Glasgow Coma Scale; include size, equality and reactivity of pupils as well as gaze (conjugate or dysconjugate); level of consciousness/mental status, motor and sensory function, verbal response every 1–4 hours to detect changes indicative of altered cerebral function.

—Note pattern and regularity of respiration if patient is not on a ventilator; monitor vital signs every 15 minutes to 1 hour; change in respiration may be a sign of increased ICP and of hypoxia and/or hypercapnia.

—Drain CSF from ventriculostomy as ordered to maintain ICP under 15–20 mm Hg.

—Watch for signs of vasospasm in patients with aneurysms (for example, depressed level of consciousness, hemiparesis. visual problems, seizures).

—Use stimulation to try to awaken a patient from coma.

—Monitor side effects of drug (for example, adenine arabinoside can alter renal function and cause fluid overload; high doses of antibiotics can cause seizures; praziquantel can increase inflammatory response and increase intracranial pressure).

EVALUATION CRITERIA

The patient

—Maintains or improves level of consciousness and motor and sensory function.
—Has vital signs within normal limits.
—Has ICP readings of 0–15 mm Hg, cerebral perfusion pressure readings greater than 50 mm Hg.

NURSING DIAGNOSIS

a. Ineffective airway clearance related to
    —Weakness, fatigue.
    —Aspiration.
    —Cranial nerve dysfunction (for example, impaired gag, swallowing, and cough reflexes).
    —Obstructed airway.
b. Ineffective breathing pattern related to
    —Altered level of consciousness.
    —Immobility.
    —Neuromuscular dysfunction or injury, demyelination of nerves.
    —Depressed respiratory effort.
c. Impaired gas exchange related to
    —Muscle paralysis.
    —Aspiration.
    —Spinal cord edema.
    —Atelectasis.
    —Infection.
    —Increased ICP.
    —Preexisting pulmonary disease.
    —Alteration in level of consciousness.

GOALS

The patient will maintain a patent airway and adequate ventilation; will be free from cyanosis and signs of respiratory distress.

INTERVENTIONS

—Monitor respiratory status continuously (vital because C1–C4 injuries to the spinal cord result in complete loss of respiratory function; injuries to C4–C5 can result in variable loss of respiratory function due to phrenic nerve involvement and loss of diaphragmatic function).

—Assess patient for changes in level of consciousness, which may indicate cerebral hypoxia.

—Monitor respiratory rate and tidal volume (a gradual decrease in tidal volume and increased respiratory rate may indicate advancing muscular weakness or paralysis).

—Monitor for signs of pulmonary infection (for example, note characteristic color, amount, tenacity of sputum).

—Monitor arterial blood gases as appropriate; consider use of ear oximeter if arterial blood gases are labile.

—Monitor vital capacity and inspiratory force to detect increasing muscle paralysis and declining respiratory effort; if vital capacity falls to about 50% of normal or there is evidence of pharyngeal paralysis, relaxed laryngeal reflexes, or increased bronchial secretions, consider elective intubation.

—Check skin color for developing cyanosis or duskiness; note any dyspnea, orthopnea, restlessness.

—Assess patient for factors that impede lung expansion (for example, abdominal distention).

—Inspect chest for symmetrical expansion, neck veins for distention.

—Assess for ability to handle secretions, signs and symptoms of pulmonary embolism or respiratory fatigue.

—Be aware that disruption in muscle innervation and tone may jeopardize the airway by relaxation of the tongue or inability to generate an effective cough to clear secretions.

—Take precautions to prevent aspiration (for example, administer tube feedings or have patient eat in upright position); maintain cuff inflation if artificial airway is in place.

—Monitor use of respiratory depressant drugs.

—Use apnea alarm system if indicated.

—Remember that even though a patient's spinal cord injury is at a level that spares the diaphragm (for example, C5), during the acute phase there may be ascending cord edema that could impair the diaphragm.

—Demonstrate to ventilator-dependent patient with a tracheostomy how to call for help by tongue-clicking or lip-smacking.

—Instruct patient and caregivers to work and troubleshoot the ventilator.

—Minimize suctioning time (that is, get in and out quickly); hyperoxygenate and hyperventilate prior to suctioning.

—Position patient on side to maintain patent airway if unresponsive or postictal.

—Assist patient with "quad coughing" if indicated.

—Enhance the patient's lung expansion and efforts to cough by elevating the head of the bed to keep the abdominal contents off the diaphragm and to facilitate normal chest expansion.

—Ensure caregivers understand when to call the doctor, what routine and preventative pulmonary care to provide.

—Discourage smoking through patient education.
—Provide oxygen therapy as indicated.
—Perform chest physiotherapy and encourage incentive spirometry as appropriate.
—Ausculate presence or absence of breath sounds; note development of adventitious sounds such as rhonchi or wheezes; increased airway resistance and/or accumulation of secretions will impede gas exchange.

EVALUATION CRITERIA

The patient

—Has clear breath sounds.
—Is free from signs of hypoxia and hypercarbia.
—Has adequate arterial blood gases.

The patient and caregiver

—Verbalize understanding of any pulmonary care and maintenance of the ventilator if the patient will be ventilator-dependent at home.
—Verbalize signs and symptoms of potential problems and report to the physician promptly.

NURSING DIAGNOSIS

Impaired physical mobility related to

—Altered level of consciousness.
—Enforced bedrest, immobilization.
—Neuromuscular deficit: paralysis, paresthesia, weakness.
—Pain.
—Motor and/or sensory deficits.
—Cognitive impairment.
—Assistive devices (for example, respirator, halo, lack of mobility aids).
—Decreased strength and endurance.
—Decreased range of motion, flexibility.
—Fatigue, weakness.

GOALS

The patient will be free from preventable complications of immobility (for example, wrist or foot drop, contractures, external rotation of hip).

INTERVENTIONS

—Prevent footdrop by using space boots on the lower extremities.
—Apply elastic stockings or mechanical deep vein thrombosis (DVT) pneu-

matic stockings on the legs of patients confined to bed; prophalactic anticoagulation may be prescribed.

—Follow measures in box below to prevent venous thrombosis, especially in patients receiving aminocaproic acid.

—Watch for side effects of drugs, such as clot formation in other parts of the body (for example, pulmonary embolus).

Prophylactic Venous Thrombosis Protocol for Spinal Cord Injuries
Goal: to prevent venous thrombosis in acute spinal cord injured patients.
1. Measure circumference of thigh and calf daily at point 20 cm below and above the upper border of the patella.
2. Apply full length (toe to groin) elastic hose; remove hose for 30 minutes every shift.
3. Keep knees slightly flexed. Do not place pads in popliteal space.
4. Place patient in Trendelenberg position (about 15°) a minimum of one hour every eight hours unless contraindicated, as in chest injury or increased intracranial pressure.
5. Range of motion to lower extremities QID per instruction of doctor or physical therapist.
6. Notify physician of:
   —Increase in thigh or calf circumference by 2 cm from one day to the next.
   —Increased temperature of any area of either lower extremity.
   —Reddened area on either extremity.
   —Complaints of pain or discomfort in those patients with sensation.

—Be alert for signs of local redness, heat, swelling in an extremity with stiffness of involved joints, which may be signs of heterotrophic ossification.

—Maintain proper spinal alignment.

—Initiate passive or active range-of-motion exercises as soon as possible to enhance circulation and prevent contractures.

—Get patient up on tilt table or mobilized as soon as possible to halt decalcification of the bones; even artificial weight bearing will prevent this complication; if patient is in a halo brace, mobilize to the chair.

—Mobilize patient slowly to minimize effects of postural hypotension.

—Monitor for signs of pulmonary infection, inability to handle secretions, pulmonary embolism, and respiratory fatigue.

—Perform chest physiotherapy (percussion and postural drainage) as indicated; encourage use of spirometry if ordered.

—Consider use of kinetic bed to help prevent pulmonary complications and other problems from immobility; remember that a kinetic bed may increase peristalsis and the patient can develop diarrhea.

—Begin prescribed bowel program upon admission.

—Avoid using bedpan under immobile patient with spinal cord injury; it may cause spinal misalignment and scrape the skin, causing an open sore.
—See box on page 214 for care of a patient in a halo brace.
—Log roll patients postoperatively; realize that this activity may be very frightening for the patient who fears turning will damage the spine.
—Progress patients slowly after cervical laminectomy by increasing the level of head elevation before sitting or dangling at the bedside.
—Provide a back brace for support during ambulation if needed for patient with a thoracic laminectomy.
—Progress patient toward ambulation over about a week's time after lumbar laminectomy.
—Counsel regarding home hospice programs that provide home nursing care, pain control, and companionship during final stages of a disease process involving increased immobility, such as brain tumor.
—Avoid taking all hope away from patients with a devastating injury such as a spinal cord injury; most patients, regardless of how long they have had their spinal cord injury, never give up all hope that they will one day be mobile again.

EVALUATION CRITERIA

The patient

—Is free of deformities developed since time of physical immobility.
—Is free from complications of immobility.
—Maintains flexibility of all joints.

NURSING DIAGNOSIS

Self-care deficit in feeding, bathing and/or hygiene, dressing and/or grooming, and toileting related to

—Altered level of consciousness.
—Neuromuscular deficit.
—Sensory-perceptual deficits: visual field cut, diminished sensation, agnosia, apraxia.
—Cognitive impairment, altered awareness of socially acceptable behavior.
—Altered behavior.
—Altered thought processes.
—Activity intolerance.
—Apathy, fatigue.
—Pain.
—Weakness or paralysis.
—Depression, frustration.
—Inability to communicate.

Care of the Patient in a Halo Brace

—Clean skull pin sites with betadine solution twice a day. There should be no crust around the sites. If there is a crust, it should be soaked with saline-saturated 4×4's.

—Check skull pin sites daily for signs of infection. If patient complains of pain at pin site, the pin may be loose and need to be torqued.

—Check bolts on the vest for finger tightness daily.

—Never move patient by bars of the vest.

—Skin under vest can be washed and dried thoroughly. A wash cloth which has been squeezed out well will not saturate the lining.

—Avoid powder under the vest.

—Check for pressure areas under vest with a flashlight daily. A pillowcase can be slipped through the vest from one side to the other. If it comes out with any serosanguinous drainage, it may indicate an area of skin breakdown.

—The halo vest liner may need to be changed if the patient has perspired heavily or dropped crumbs down the front. This liner change may be done by the physician or a nursing halo team member.

—The halo device limits the visual field by restricting head movement. Prism glasses or a hand mirror may help overcome this.

—If the patient complains of difficulty swallowing, it should be reported to the physician, as the neck may be out of alignment.

—Assist patient in ambulating or getting up until he is used to the weight of the vest to prevent falling.

—Know how to remove anterior vest in case the need to get to the chest to do CPR arises.

—Instruct patient to report any new numbness or tingling in his arms or fingers.

—A patient's hair may be shampooed, either by using a shampoo board or by placing the patient on a cart with his head off the end, strapped to the cart. Do not use metal equipment to wash the hair because when it hits the metal parts of the halo, it vibrates and is very irritating to the patient. Assure that no water drains under the vest onto the lining.

—Be aware that patients may have psychological after-effects of halo traction. The patient may believe that his paralysis and immobility are a result of confinement in the halo brace, rather than a result of the injury. Or he may believe that once the spine has healed the deficit will be gone. The patient develops a false sense of hopefulness that once the halo is removed, be will not be disabled. When this does not occur, severe depression and delayed reaction to the injury may be seen.

—Keep hair around posterior skull pins clipped in order to see the sites, one-half inch in diameter.

—Avoid using a donut pad under a patient's head or any part of his body, for it has a tourniquet effect, cutting off blood supply to the center area.

—Use side-to-side weight shifts. A forward shift may cause the patient to fall because of the weight of the vest.

—Encourage prone sleeping for the following reasons:
  • It aids skin inspection.

- It takes pressure off scapulae.
- It stimulates circulatory exchange.
- It aids in prevention of formation of renal calculi due to urinary stasis.
- It minimizes gastrointestinal complications brought on by stasis.

—Use position pads, thick enough to support the upright bars and elevate the patient's face. Use a pillow under the chest for support and pressure equalization. The neck curvature may be supported by a soft pillow. Avoid placing pressure, such as from a pillow, directly on the halo ring.

GOALS

The patient will meet self-care needs; will be able to perform a schedule of activities appropriate to condition and mental readiness.

INTERVENTIONS

—Determine patient's ability to perform activities of daily living; assess response to self-care activities to determine tolerance.
—Establish means of communication for patient to express needs (for example, alphabet charts, one eyeblink or squeeze of hand for "yes," two for "no").
—If patient has a visual field cut, arrange bed in the room so patient will be able to see people approaching.
—Place call light on nonparetic side.
—Approach patient from side with good vision.
—Teach patient to visually scan the environment.
—Begin rehabilitation as soon as patient is stable medically; planning conferences with family, physical and occupational therapists, speech therapist, nurse, physician, dietician, social worker, psychologist, and sometimes the patient, too, makes everyone aware of the goals for the patient and how to deal with current issues.
—Allow for adequate rest periods between activities to avoid fatigue and frustration.
—Praise the patient for good performance in doing a skill; stress the positive and give encouragement for gains in self-care activities.
—Explain to patient what has happened to him and reassure that he is being cared for.
—Explain procedure or tasks to patient before starting them; especially if an agnosia (that is, failure to recognize and identify objects or configurations through a sense otherwise intact) is evident; a patient may not know what to do with a comb or toothbrush placed in his hand.
—Repeat tasks such as feeding or dressing to reduce the apraxia (inability to perform a learned movement voluntarily); families can help with this repetition.

—Encourage expression of feelings about inability to do self-care tasks or about satisfaction of relearning self-care competency.

—Obtain necessary assistive devices to enable patient to function maximally (for example, hand splints, adaptive silverware, raised toilet seat).

—Introduce new skill slowly, providing uses, and allowing patient opportunity to practice until it becomes habitual.

EVALUATION CRITERIA

The patient

—Appears well-groomed, clean, comfortable, well-nourished and hydrated.

The patient and family

—Demonstrate complete care.

19

Sleep-Rest Pattern

The sleep-rest pattern focuses on the patient's normal patterns of sleep, rest, and relaxation.

The nursing diagnosis that is most useful for patients experiencing neurologic injury or dysfunction and associated with this functional health pattern is sleep pattern disturbance.

Sleep Pattern Disturbance. Patients with neurologic impairment are frequently hospitalized for a time as a result of the condition, and a subsequent disruption in sleep pattern occurs. Hallucinations, pain, and fatigue may also disrupt normal sleep patterns. A patient in the hospital setting may have great difficulty sleeping. Strange noises and procedures may be going on during the night as well as during the day. The bed may feel strange. The patient may have pain and anxiety. Many issues contribute to a patient becoming sleep-deprived at a time when rest may be very important.

NURSING DIAGNOSIS

Sleep pattern disturbance related to

—Hospital environment.
—Pain.
—Anxiety.
—Disorientation.
—Post-traumatic syndrome.

GOALS

The patient will establish an effective sleep pattern.

INTERVENTIONS

—Find out what the patient's bedtime rituals are and maintain them during hospitalization; take a sleep activity history.
—Assess the source of the disturbance.

—Provide a quiet environment for sleep and turn out the overhead lights whenever possible.

—Tell patient that you will not be interrupting him so he can sleep for a designated period.

—Refrain from equating sleep with the absence of pain; analgesia may need to be administered around the clock to keep pain from getting out of control.

—Inquire regarding the quality of sleep the patient obtains, and what might make it better; review patient's use of home sleep aids and their effectiveness.

—Refresh the patient before sleep (for example, a backrub, warm milk, soft music).

—Maintain wakefulness during the day so the patient doesn't sleep all day.

—Teach relaxation techniques (for example, self-hypnosis, biofeedback).

—Discourage intake of stimulants (for example, coffee, tea, chocolate, cola) before rest period.

—Allow patient to discuss any concerns to possibly reduce his psychological stress; provide emotional support; reassure with factual information.

—Encourage quiet activities such as reading before sleep.

EVALUATION CRITERIA

The patient

—Receives 6 hours of uninterrupted sleep at night.

—Sleeps at night and is awake most of the day.

—Verbalizes that he feels rested.

—Is free from dark circles under eyes, frequent yawning, expressionless face, disorientation, irritability.

—Verbalizes satisfaction with sleep pattern.

—Verbalizes reduced fatigue.

CHAPTER **20**

Cognitive-Perceptual Pattern

The cognitive-perceptual pattern covers the functioning of sensory modes, and the interpretation of stimuli—pain—in particular. Impairment of the nervous system may disrupt sensory and motor transmissions or influence the way a signal is interpreted by the brain.

The nursing diagnoses that are most useful for patients experiencing neurologic injury or dysfunction and associated with the cognitive-perceptual functional health pattern include alteration in comfort—pain, alteration in thought processes, knowledge deficit, sensory-perceptual alteration, and unilateral neglect.

Alteration in Comfort: Pain. Neurologic injuries or pathology may result in severe pain. Sensation of pain has different meanings for different individuals. Head pain, in particular, may be stressful and cause a person to believe the cause of the pain is far worse than the actual etiology. In addition to direct neurologic trauma, there are often coexisting injuries that may also result in pain and headache.

Alteration in Thought Processes. Cognitive disarrangement after neurologic insult is common, especially following direct head trauma. Thought processes are altered, resulting in poor judgment, disorientation, inability to solve problems, inpulsiveness, short attention span, loss of social inhibitions, egocentricity with a lack of sensitivity to other people's needs, problems with sequencing of tasks, and many other deficits. The thinking process of someone with head trauma may not be based on reality, but on a misinterpretation of the environment. Sometimes the alterations in thought processes are transient and improve with time. Other times, even with specific cognitive retraining, the individual requires some degree of lifelong supervision.

Knowledge Deficit. Patients without adequate knowledge about their disorder or deficit may be less compliant with their therapy and be far more anxious than necessary. When the patient is cognitively impaired, the caregivers must be given the information, so they understand the implications of the impairment and the needs of the patient.

Sensory-Perceptual Alteration. Neurologic injury may result in altered sensory reception and transmission and integration of stimuli, so the interpretation of environmental stimuli is inaccurate. Perception of reality is altered. Other causes of altered perception may include factors such as sleep-deprivation, ICU psychosis, stress, pain, anxiety, or impaired ability to communicate or respond to environmental stimuli. There may also be physiologic reasons that sensory reception cannot occur, as with spinal cord injury.

Unilateral Neglect. Patients with unilateral neglect usually fail to respond to the environmental stimuli on the contralateral side to the brain injury. There may be concomitant hemianopia, hemianesthesia, or hemiparesis. Unilateral neglect is often associated with right hemisphere lesions, usually of the right inferior parietal lobe, which is responsible for sensory association and integrating multimodality (visual, tactile, and auditory) stimuli. Patients who show inattention or neglect to one side of their bodies and to one-half of the environment can exhibit behavior that is confusing or frightening to families.

NURSING DIAGNOSIS

Alteration in comfort: pain related to

—Vasodilatation of cerebral vessels.
—Intracranial lesions, trauma.
—Increased intracranial pressure.
—Irritation and/or inflammation of muscles, joints, meninges.
—Response to therapy and/or diagnostic procedures.
—Surgery.
—Trauma.
—Positioning.
—Photophobia.
—Stress.
—Pressure on nerves.

GOALS

The patient will experience an increase in comfort; will exhibit relaxed facial expression; will regain baseline vital signs.

INTERVENTIONS

—Assess for factors that decrease pain tolerance (for example, fear, fatigue, monotony); reduce or eliminate factors; acknowledge presence of pain and your desire to minimize it.
—Give medication as ordered in a timely manner; monitor effectiveness;

small scheduled doses of analgesia may keep the pain under better control than giving it only after the pain has become severe.

—Instruct the patient in the timing of taking prescribed medications; for example, teach to use ergotamine derivatives at the first sign of headache; caution that if the ergot drugs are used too frequently, without several days of interruption as recommended, a medication headache cycle called rebounding can occur.

—Explain the causes of the pain if possible; how long it will last and what will help reduce it.

—Observe for favorable response to therapy; assess patient's willingness and ability to participate in noninvasive methods of controlling pain.

—Help determine what relieves and what aggravates pain for the patient; help patient to eliminate or minimize trigger factors such as coughing and straining that may aggravate a headache.

—Give reassurance; communicate your acceptance of the patient's pain and response to it.

—Teach relaxation and distraction techniques (see Table 20.1).

Table 20.1.
Pain Management Techniques

Relaxation Techniques

Purpose:	Reduce anxiety
	Reduce skeletal muscle tension
	Interrupt cycle of increased pain, anxiety, muscle tension, despair
	Provide distraction from pain
	Combat fatigue
	Increase ability to cope with intensity of pain
Means:	Warm bath
	Massage
	Back rub
	Soft music
	Rhythmic breathing exercises that focus attention away from pain

Distraction Techniques

Purpose:	Focus attention on stimuli other than the pain, forcing pain to the periphery of awareness
	May tire patient because of energy required to perform them, so use for brief periods
Means:	Counting objects
	Guided imagery
	Singing
	Audio and/or video tapes

—Approach patient unhurriedly and allow patient to verbalize feelings about his own perception of the pain, which may vary with different cultural, ethnic and social influences.

—Provide cutaneous stimulation (for example, massage, heat, cold, vibration), which is a combination of distraction, relaxation, and therapeutic touch.

—Teach the patient stress management techniques to facilitate coping with the pain.

—Keep lights dim and the environment quiet to allow for adequate rest, especially after an analgesic is administered.

—If the pain is related to intracranial pressure, facilitate venous drainage from head by elevating the head of the bed 30 degrees and have the patient keep head in neutral alignment.

—Prepare the patient for a painful experience; for example, explain preoperatively what to expect in the postoperative phase.

EVALUATION CRITERIA

The patient

—Verbalizes relief of pain.
—Identifies factors that influence pain.
—Demonstrates use of pain relief measures, including self-administration of medications appropriately and relaxation techniques.

NURSING DIAGNOSIS

Alteration in thought processes related to
—Increased intracranial pressure.
—Metabolic and/or electrolyte disturbances.
—Side effects of medications.
—Sleep deprivation.
—Perceptual alterations.
—Cognitive deficits.
—Cerebral pathology (for example, area of brain infarction, encephalopathy, contusion).
—Altered level of consciousness.
—Posttraumatic syndrome.

GOALS

The patient will be oriented to time, place, and person; will voluntarily interact with others in socially appropriate ways; will remain free from injury.

INTERVENTIONS

—Help establish a means of communication, either verbal, written, or using one and two eyeblinks or hand squeezes to indicate "yes" and "no."

—Repeat who the caregiver is because of deficit in recognizing people.

—Label drawers, bathroom, clothes, and other items in the Alzheimer patient's environment.

—"Get patient's attention before speaking; say name, wait for eye contact, speak slowly, distinctly, and loud enough to be heard; turn off radio, television, and shut out other distractions.

—Use a voice tone that indicates sincerity, sensitivity, respect, and acceptance.

—Give patient choices when possible, but avoid meaningless, unnecessary changes (for example, in roommate, decor, routines), which are often upsetting to patients with organic brain syndrome.

—Answer questions repeatedly as necessary, using short, simple sentences; reinforce verbal communication with gestures; build on the sensible statements of the patient to strengthen reality-based conversation.

—Provide orientation to time/place/person every hour; use clocks, calendars, signs, pictures, and written reminders; put patient's picture and name (in big letters) on the door to room and on bed.

—Use concrete symbols (for example, photographs, tangible creations, and products) of patient's past to strengthen and reassure patient's sense of continuity of self (now threatened with brain deterioration).

—Encourage to review past in order to remember and savor happy events, friendships, trips, achievements; even if content of reminiscences produces sadness, resentment, or angry outbursts, there is value in ventilating and working through those feelings before changing the subject to a more pleasant one.

—Utilize volunteers to visit or write letters for patient, to show films, hold concerts, or entertain, to take patients for outings of grounds or in neighborhood.

—Arrange for some kind of meaningful occupational therapy (e.g., simple repetitive activities such as clipping coupons, packaging items, stuffing envelopes)." (Caine & Bufalino, 1987: 168–169)

—Minimize memory impairment by repetition, having patient write down important facts if possible, and carrying this information with him in a notebook.

—Give empathy regarding the frustration of being unable to communicate, remember, or perform; distraction from the frustration may be appropriate if it interferes with daily performance.

—Use brief teaching periods when expecting the patient to learn something new because attention span is brief; do teaching in an area with minimal surrounding distractions.

—Instruct family that patient's altered thought processes may affect the ability to follow commands, both mentally understanding the command and voluntarily initiating the motor response.

—Structure environment and daily schedule to help in the process of cognitive retraining.

—Ensure safety because judgment maay be affected and there may be impaired ability to reason and solve problems; poor judgment may put the patient at risk for self-injury.

—Instruct family that egocentricity is common after head injury, that this is a sequella of the injury; prepare the family for feeling they are living with a stranger, because the patient's personality can change drastically.

—Warn family members of the possibility of inappropriate social behavior, inappropriate affect, hallucinations, delusions, and altered sleep patterns.

—Refer the family and patient to the Head Injury Foundation for group sessions and educational material.

—Relate to the patient on an adult level, not on a parent-child level.

—Divide tasks into multiple simple steps.

—Approach patient in unhurried manner; allow time for thought comprehension.

—Reduce physical discomforts that might interfere with cognitive function.

—Correct misinterpreted messages immediately.

—Encourage decision-making when possible.

—Give explicit directions when asking patient to perform a task.

—Correct vision and hearing deficits if present; sensory deprivation from vision and hearing loss may add to the patient's confusion.

—Assure adequate lighting in the environment to reduce confusion.

—Use distraction with patients who become combative.

—Honor the patient's agenda, that is, the wandering, confused, restless, and combative behavior that may be seen in patients who have a plan of action that counteracts reality; it lessens confusion, anxiety, and sense of isolation, and saves family or nurses time.

—Monitor television shows patients with Alzheimer's disease watch (television violence may be confused with reality and cause patient to become agitated).

—Encourage patient to wear identification band with name, address, phone number, and name of physician to contact; ensure it reads "memory impaired."

—Listen with tolerance (the same story or complaint may be verbalized repeatedly).

—Be sure medications are given under supervision to ensure that patient gets the proper dose of the proper drugs and does not forget to take them.

EVALUATION CRITERIA

The patient

—Communicates needs.
—Participates in some decisions about activities of daily living.
—Demonstrates appropriate social behavior.
—Is oriented to time, place, and person.

NURSING DIAGNOSIS

Knowledge deficit regarding

—Diagnosis.
—Treatment.
—Expected outcomes.
—Precipitating factors.
—Specific options available.
—Signs and symptoms of complications.
—Side effects of treatment and medications.
—Energy conservation.

GOALS

The patient and family will verbalize implications of the impairment; will follow through with instructions; will verbalize and demonstrate an understanding of the treatment regimen, expected outcomes, and life-style adjustments.

INTERVENTIONS

—Determine patient's and family's present knowledge and perception of the neurologic problem; establish learning needs of patient and family as a baseline for a teaching plan.
—Implement teaching plan using the following principles of teaching and learning:

   • Note level of anxiety and lower if necessary; mild to moderate level is ideal for learning; high anxiety impairs concentration, memory recall, and ability to listen.
   • Consider the timing of any teaching that is done; during an early acute phase of illness, patient may be too concerned about survival to be able to retain specific instructions.
   • Provide a quiet, uninterrupted environment with privacy to do the teaching.

- Provide instructions in small amounts at a time, especially if the patient's attention span is limited.
- Ask patient and family what they want to learn about first; if one issue is of great concern to them at a particular time, they will not be able to give their full attention to the topic you have chosen to talk about.
- Create an accepting and supportive environment for the patient and family to ask questions.
- Use repetition in giving information; use different words with the same meaning.
- Have patient and family reiterate information and/or demonstrate a procedure that has been taught to be sure they understand it; correct misconceptions as needed.

—Use forms of behavior modification to get the appropriate performance from a patient who is cognitively impaired; teach family to follow same techniques at home if indicated.
—Provide patient and family with community resources such as support groups or educational resources.
—Instruct myasthenic patient in importance of taking the prescribed medication on a regular schedule; educate about side effects of anticholinesterase drug and how to minimize them (for example, taking the drug with food or milk will minimize GI side effects).
—Instruct patients with T7 or higher level of spinal cord injury about signs or symptoms and treatment of autonomic dysreflexia.
—Instruct a patient with a seizure disorder about drug therapy prescribed by physician and factors that may trigger a seizure (for example, abrupt withdrawl of medication, alcohol, fatigue, excessive stress, menstruation, fever, large amounts of caffeine).
—Emphasize common side effects of anticonvulsant (for example, blood dyscrasias, anemia, rash or skin eruptions, drowsiness, GI irritation, and gingival problems; provide guidelines to deal with side effects.
—Consider a home evaluation visit prior to discharge or weekend pass so patient and family can identify obstacles in the home situation.

EVALUATION CRITERIA

The patient and family

—Correctly demonstrate procedures taught.
—Ask appropriate questions.
—Demonstrate understanding of the impairment.
—Verbalize necessary life-style changes.

NURSING DIAGNOSIS

Sensory-perceptual alteration related to

—Altered level of consciousness.
—Impaired sensation, sensory deficits.
—Inability to integrate and interpret environmental stimuli.
—Restricted and/or unfamiliar environment.
—Side effects of medications.
—Disorientation.
—Impaired communication skills.

GOALS

The patient will regain and maintain sensory equilibrium; will be able to interpret appropriately incoming stimuli; will demonstrate optimal contact with reality.

INTERVENTION

—Protect patient from injury since patient may not feel sensation of pain, heat, or body position.
—Provide stimuli for the patient but prevent sensory overload; include some familiar sounds, such as family's voices on tape or in person.
—Allow for adequate sleep; alter lighting and reduce auditory stimuli to help reestablish normal circadian sleep patterns.
—Monitor level of sensation (sharp and dull) and report any increase in sensory deficit.
—Provide orientation aids such as clocks and calendars.
—Explain strange noises in the environment to allow for accurate interpretation by the patient.
—Patch eyes on a rotating basis to allow for some clear visual input if diplopia is present.
—Encourage family members to touch and talk to patient to keep patient oriented; help them understand that touching does not hurt the patient.
—Explain procedures prior to initiating them.
—Help prevent misinterpretation of information by monitoring conversation around bedside.
—Note and make cards of perceptual deficits and place at bedside to alert all caregivers (for example, "Patient cannot speak").
—Describe the patient's environment and provide conversation to the unconscious patient as if he were awake.
—Apply coma-stimulation techniques to try to awaken a patient from coma (see box below).

Coma Stimulation Techniques

Purpose: To awaken patient from coma.

—Use stimulation to all the senses.
- Have patient smell a fragrance, such as coffee.
- Turn on radio or television intermittently. Continuous auditory stimulation becomes background noise and is not paid attention.
- Familiar family voices talking to the patient may be useful, whether the family is there in person or whether it is a tape recording.
- Stimulate sense of touch by rubbing ice bags or a heating pad over different areas of the patient's body.
- Use further sensory stimulation by putting textured material such as velcro or velvet in patient's hands.
- Stimulate taste with lemon and glycerin swabs or other distinct tastes, such as peppermint, in patient's mouth.
- Stimulate sense of sight by placing colorful balloons or familiar pictures within eyesight.
- Place patient in areas of high traffic or activity intermittently for visual and auditory stimulation.

—It has been said by some patients who have awakened from comatose states that coma is a comfortable, quiet state. The patient wants to be left alone and undisturbed. Stimulation is noxious to this state and may cause the patient to want to wake up and stop the disturbance. Otherwise there may be no desire to awaken from the comfortable state of unconsciousness.

—The nurse is never sure how much perception an unconcious patient has. He may be perceiving most of what is happening in the environment, but there may be no motor connection to show others that he is perceiving. Because we can never be sure, we should tell patients what we are going to do to them prior to doing any procedure. In not doing this, we dehumanize our nursing care of these patients.

—Monitor what is said around the bedside. Nothing should be said that would not be said to the patient were he completely awake.

—Encourage families to help in providing care and stimulation of patients when possible and appropriate. Help them understand that they are not going to hurt the patient if they touch him.

EVALUATION CRITERIA

The patient

—Is aware of environment as much as level of consciousness will permit.
—Obtains adequate rest.

NURSING DIAGNOSIS

Unilateral neglect related to

—Neurologic illness/damage.
—Trauma/brain injury.
—Stroke.
—Cerebral tumor.

GOALS

The patient will acknowledge the affected side; will perform range-of-motion and/or other therapies on affected side; will identify safety hazards in environment.

INTERVENTIONS

—Make patient aware of the side he is ignoring by reminding patient of that side and where that extremity is in space.
—Encourage touching of the side to which the patient shows inattention; encourage patient to rub and massage extremity, especially during bathing; have patient watch his arm or leg as he strokes it.
—Provide for patient's safety (for example, patients may need a Posey jacket restraint at night because they forget they have a deficit and may try to get up and walk to the bathroom on a paralyzed limb).
—Teach to scan the environment visually with head so the total area is perceived, to overcome the side neglected.
—Use behavior modification programs to help remediate some of the behaviors asociated with hemiinattention; constantly cue patient to the environment.
—Instruct patient to keep affected extremity in view and to take care around sources of heat or cold.
—Place patient in a room so unaffected side is facing the central activity in the room.
—Approach patient from unaffected side.
—Place patient's food tray toward unaffected side; position bed with unaffected side toward the door.
—Encourage patient to perform activities of daily living such as shaving and brushing teeth in front of a mirror and with supervision.
—Use verbal instructions for patients with right hemispheric lesions.
—Place patient's unaffected side near a wall when working with affected extremities to minimize distraction and help focus attention on affected extremities.
—Minimize visual distractions when providing care or working with patient.
—Keep the room well-lighted.
—Position a full-length mirror in patient's environment.
—Make family aware of patient's deficits, especially since they may not be readily apparent, to help family better understand patient's frustrations.

—Position call light, bedside stand, telephone, television on unaffected side.

EVALUATION CRITERIA

The patient

—Is free from self-harm.
—Uses affected side as much as physically possible.

SUGGESTED READINGS

Caine R, Bufalino P: *Nursing Care Planning Guides for Adults.* Baltimore, Williams & Wilkins, 1987.
Frey V, Hockett C, Moist G: *Nursing Diagnosis Care Plans.* Baltimore, Williams & Wilkins, 1986.
Neal M, Cohen P, Reighley J: *Nursing Care Planning Guides, Set 6.* Baltimore, Williams & Wilkins, 1986.

CHAPTER 21

Self-perception/ Self-concept Pattern

The self-perception/self concept pattern combines information regarding the way a patient sees self, one's own abilities (cognitive, affective, and physical), and general worth or value. The patient with a neurologic impairment experiences a major assalt to his sense of self; nurses must recognize disruptions in self-perception and take appropriate action.

The nursing diagnoses that are most useful for patients experiencing neurologic injury or dysfunction and associated with the functional health pattern self-concept/self-perception include anxiety; disturbance in self-concept: body image, self-esteem, role performance, personal identity; and powerlessness.

Anxiety. Neuromuscular illness or injuries pose a threat to the patient and family. The condition may be temporary with no long-term changes required, or it may be permanent, requiring life-long modifications of the patient and family. Temporary anxiety may be brought about by postoperative pain. The pain is distressful for only a brief period of time, and then it resolves. No long-term adjustments are necessary. On the other hand, pain caused by an inoperable brain tumor may cause stress and anxiety in the patient and family over a long period of time. If the person with the brain tumor is the family's bread winner, he may no longer be able to work, may be hospitalized intermittently, and may no longer be able to perform in his previous role within the family and the community. The patient or a family member may develop severe anxiety in response to the uncertainties brought on by the condition, treatments, or life-style modifications.

Disturbance in Self-concept. Neurologic deficits frequently lead to some disturbance in the self-concept. If the deficit is visible, such as necessitating being in a wheelchair or use of other aids, the self-concept may be more altered than an invisible or minimal deficit, such as a mild speech disorder. Head-injured patients may not have a visible impairment, but they and their family know they are not quite the same person as they were before the injury. Subtle deficits, such as impaired judgment, difficulty with decision making, problem solving, and a short attention span may not be visible to outsiders, but may actually incapacitate a head-injured victim. Regardless of the severity of the altered self-concept, it is often an issue that needs to be addressed, and the patient may need some help working through the process of accepting a new or altered self-concept.

Powerlessness. Powerlessness may be related to a life situation, approaching death, or to a physical loss. It is feeling that efforts are useless and ineffective. The perception of no control may be very accurate in some situations, or it may be exaggerated in others.

NURSING DIAGNOSIS

Anxiety related to

—Uncertainty of timing of seizures.
—Public stigma.
—Uncertain impact of neurologic condition on lifestyle.
—Uncertain outcomes.

GOALS

The patient will recognize own anxiety; will take steps to reduce anxiety; will achieve and maintain a functional level.

INTERVENTIONS

—Be aware that anxiety is contagious; stay calm, give valid reassurance and reinforce positive behavior.
—Identify the level of anxiety (for example, mild, moderate, severe); monitor functional capabilities.
—Identify stressors and precipating factors.
—Encourage expression of feelings, concerns, anxieties, and frustrations.
—Recognize signs of increasing anxiety; keep anxiety from escalating by providing consistent care and brief, factual information as needed.
—Speak simply, use easily understood language in a calm, modulated voice.
—Explore methods to reduce stress; role play if appropriate.
—Identify previously used coping strategies (both successes and failures) and alleviating factors that can be instituted to decrease anxiety.
—Do not contribute to or support maladaptive behaviors; maintain a firm, consistent approach with the patient. An example of maladaptive behavior might be a quadriplegic making plans to return to work as a construction worker. Without taking away all hope of recovery, we should at least introduce other options that would be available to him. We can also focus the patient on the present situation, and stress the importance of therapy now.

—Introduce and practice relaxation techniques (for example, breathing exercises, visualization, guided imagery).

—Prioritize care to assure that immediate needs are met; teach family members to prioritize. For example, urge the family of a head-injured patient to participate in reorientation and behavior modification techniques rather than focusing on the patient's previous plans for college.

—Administer medications as ordered; monitor effectiveness. If certain drugs are not effective, others may be.

—Lend perspective about the situation to widen the perceptual field and correct distortions. A patient or family may be stuck on the fact that the patient has a devastating neurologic deficit. Options for what the patient *can* do may be pointed out. Added information about a disorder or disease may help correct mistaken ideas held by patient or family.

EVALUATION CRITERIA

The patient

—Identifies anxious behaviors and precipitating factors.
—Implements techniques to decrease anxiety.

The patient and family

—Recognize behaviors indicating anxiety.
—List at least two methods of reducing anxiety.

NURSING DIAGNOSIS

Disturbance in self-concept: body image, self-esteem, role performance, personal identity related to

—Altered body structure or function.
—Inability to perform activities with previous level of success.
—Loss of independence.
—Feelings of powerlessness due to immobility.
—Role changes.
—Physical changes.

GOALS

The patient will make changes in lifestyle to cope with new self-image; will adapt to a chronic condition involving pain, decreased physical activity, some loss of independence and performance; will achieve maximal independence within physical limits.

INTERVENTIONS

—"Encourage patient to talk about impact of disability on self-image ("Other people in your situation sometimes feel their body is useless or unworkable. What is it like for you?") ("You seem sad today—what's going on?")

—Acknowledge and accept what patient says; do not deny or invalidate feelings expressed.

—Assess and discuss with patient his/her strengths and capabilities.

—Use humor and laughter to lend perspective and to facilitate acceptance of condition.

—Assess patient's readiness to undertake new tasks; intervene, if necessary, before the patient becomes frustrated or discouraged.

—Encourage and praise patient's willingness to learn new tasks.

—Be supportive in pointing out appropriate areas of control for the patient.

- Give patient time to prepare and signal the nurse when ready to begin an activity.
- Allow patient to choose the time of treatment and the order in which ADL are performed.
- Create positive outlets for aggression and frustrations (for example, punching bags, yelling out of earshot, crying).
- Accept matter-of-factly those patient behaviors that reflect a struggle with dependence-independence:

  —Extremes in behavior prior to achieving a satisfactory resolution.
  —The need to regain control of self and environment by becoming demanding and manipulative.

—Assist patient to express feelings of powerlessness and helplessness concerning immobility.

—Anticipate needs and provide a safe, secure environment to minimize anxiety and to develop trust of the nurse.

—Provide opportunity for patient to have choices about food, clothing, activities, and to be self-directing, and develop new skills.

—Foster open communication between patient and significant other.

—Act as a sounding board for family members to verbalize worries and concerns.

—Discourage inappropriate sexual flirtations by patient toward the nurse without undermining patient's self-confidence.

—Incorporate the needs of the family into the plan of care; prepare the family for the changing behavior of the patient.

—Prepare the patient for the loss of role and altered patterns of functioning in the family.

—Minimize separation and alienation of patient from the family by openly discussing with patient and family the anticipated changed family structure.

—Provide phones at bedside or wheelchair height in halls to facilitate frequent communication with friends and family.
—Schedule family conferences to provide program information, to allow questions and expressions of everyone's concerns.
—Explore how patient expects it to be at home; encourage patient to mentally "practice" own part in the changes." (Neal, Cohen, and Reighley, 1986:113–114).
—Discuss reentering the social world with any problems that may present ("Tell me how you will handle it the first time you go out socially with a friend.")

EVALUATION CRITERIA

The patient

—Verbalizes feelings regrading implications of disability.
—Describes factors that affect self-esteem and confidence.
—Is involved in self-care to degree possible.

NURSING DIAGNOSIS

Powerlessness related to

—Alteration in body image.
—Grave prognosis.
—Imposed immobility.
—Loss of ability to walk.
—Perceived lack of control over disease treatment.

GOALS

The patient will acknowledge feelings of powerlessness; will demonstrate the ability to identify and make choices concerning own health care; will demonstrate positive adaptation to hospitalization and impaired mobility.

INTERVENTIONS

—Determine degree of insight that the patient and family have into the problem; identify beliefs concerning control issues.
—Ensure patient and family have accurate information; give anticipatory guidance to help prepare for events.
—Explore available options with the patient; explore how the problem and how treatment will affect patient's life.
—Mobilize and utilize support systems.

—Evaluate strengths; give patient as much responsibility as can be handled.

—"Assist patient in setting realistic goals and defining the steps to be taken to achieve expected outcome.

—Identify factors contributing to the present state of helplessness and suggest alternatives.

—Encourage patient's verbalization of feelings of helplessness, hopelessness, frustration, and anxiety.

—Reiterate to patient, "You do have some control; these are some of your choices; let's talk about the probable outcome of each."

—Modify the environment to increase patient control (for example, put call light in reach; decrease waiting time for treatments, meals, etc.; inform patient of time schedule)." (Frey, Hockett and Moist, 1986:104) ("Tell me what time you would like your bath, rest time, so we can develop a daily schedule of activities").

EVALUATION CRITERIA

The patient

—Makes decisions regarding care as appropriate.

—Experiences an increase in personal power.

—Verbalizes needs and wants.

—Actively participates in decision making.

SUGGESTED READINGS

Frey V, Hockett C and Moist G: *Nursing Diagnosis Care Plans*. Baltimore, Williams & Wilkins, 1986.

Neal M, Cohen P, and Reighley J: *Nursing Care Planning Guides. Set 6*, Baltimore, Williams & Wilkins, 1986.

CHAPTER 22

Role-Relationship Pattern

The role-relationship pattern focuses attention on the patient's actual or perceived relationships with others and the roles assumed. Effective communication is a major influence in maintaining quality relationships. Satisfaction or dissatisfaction with relationships, roles, and resposibilities will influence an individual's life and health. Neurologic impairments may result in physical, psychosocial and/or cognitive changes that disrupt the patient's and family's normal roles, routines, and responsibilities.

The nursing diagnoses that are most useful for patients experiencing neurologic injury or dysfunction and associated with the functional health pattern role-relationship include alteration in family processes; grieving; impaired verbal communication; and impaired social interaction, social isolation.

Alteration in Family Processes. When one member of a family becomes the victim of an illness or impairment the other family members must often make numerous adjustments, either on a temporary or a permanent basis. Roles within the family often change dramatically. The family decision-making process may also need to change. The new focus of the family is on the person with the impairment, rather than on usual activities of interest.

Grieving. Patients may grieve for loss of some bodily function, (for example, vision or mobility, or loss of a limb or some body change). Anticipatory grief may occur when there is fear of a loss or fear of death. There is a normal emotional progression of the grieving process, but it varies somewhat with each individual with regard to the length of time spent in each stage. There may also be grieving of patient or family over a material loss or loss of role.

Impaired Verbal Communication. Impaired verbal communication in the neurologically impaired population is not infrequent. Paralysis of nerves or muscles or cerebral damage may influence verbalization. Artificial airways (endotracheal tube or tracheostomy) prevent vocalization. Those who are cognitively impaired may have vocalization, but the content of the communication may be confused or inappropriate.

Impaired Social Interaction, Social Isolation. Patients with impaired sppech or communication may retreat from social interactions. The same is true of other patients with a more visible neurologic problem. Patients may avoid the social stigma by isolating themselves. Depression over an unpleasant disgnosis may also lessen social interactions.

NURSING DIAGNOSIS

Alteration in family processes related to

—Diagnosis.
—Realization that the patient is not the same person he was (for example, memory less, poor judgment and problem-solving ability, inability to reason or calculate or communicate, altered personality).
—Impaired ability of patient to meet self-care needs, role responsibilities.
—Financial burden.
—Fear.
—Helplessness.

GOALS

The family will learn to adapt to new roles necessitated by the impaired patient; will exhibit functional behaviors in present crisis.

INTERVENTIONS

—Identify the precipitating event (for example, illness, trauma) that has caused the crisis; determine the impact on the family; articulate the problem clearly and validate with all family members.
—Explore strengths and resources with the family members; utilize internal and external family resources as available and appropriate.
—Facilitate ventilation of feelings of helplessness, anger, sorrow and confusion; give empathy and support.
—Refer to outside resources such as support groups and/or social services resources for financial assistance.
—Lend perspective and give feedback to assist family in viewing problem from one another's point of view.
—Be alert to verbal and nonverbal cues indicating withdrawl of one family member or hostility of one toward another; encourage family members to accept feelings of others as valid and to express own feelings and needs.
—Assure that the family has accurate information about the patient and his situation; correct any misinformation or misunderstanding.
—Provide opportunities for family to participate in problem solving; teach how to explore alternatives and evaluate probable outcomes.

EVALUATION CRITERIA

The family

—Demonstrates effective problem-solving techniques.
—Demonstrates effective communication within family unit.
—Verbalizes satisfaction with current situation.

NURSING DIAGNOSIS

Anticipatory grieving and grieving related to

—Perceived losses: neuromuscular function, cognitive abilities, role, previous lifestyle, partner, family member.
—Irreversibility or progression of the condition.
—Prospect of death or disability.

GOALS

The patient and family will verbalize feelings about actual or anticipated loss; will move through the grieving process.

INTERVENTIONS

—Identify patient and family perceptions of the loss and meaning of loss.
—Observe nonverbal cues that may indicate some feeling other than what is being verbalized.
—Assess how patient is handling the anticipated loss, what coping behaviors are evident.
—Encourage and promote verbalization of feelings; acknowledge that the feelings are normal and expected under the circumstances.
—Help patient and family identify strengths and resources that may help them through this time; offer additional resources or options if appropriate.
—Encourage patient and family to focus on one day at a time initially; long-term projecting may seem too overwhelming at first.
—Provide simple accurate information about diagnosis and care; include an explanation of the grieving process.
—Provide realistic feedback and lend perceptions required to correct distortions.
—Provide information on support groups and outside resources.
—Identify specific problems anticipated by the loss and assist patient in recognizing alternatives.
—Be aware that the family may grieve for the patient who is not the same person now that dementia or cognitive dysfunction is present.

EVALUATION CRITERIA

The patient/family

—Expresses feelings.
—Begins to progress through recognized stages of grieving.

NURSING DIAGNOSIS

Impaired verbal communication related to

—Intubation.
—Tracheostomy.
—Neurologic deficit, brain damage.
—Cranial nerve paresis or paralysis.
—Dysarthia.
—Impaired breathing.
—Disorientation, confusion.

GOALS

The patient will communicate by some method.

INTERVENTIONS

—Talk to the patient as an adult, not as a child; speak at an ordinary conversation level; reduce extraneous room sounds.
—Set up some method for the patient to communicate; try vocalization, writing, pointing to letters of the alphabet, pointing to pictures of what he may need, eyeblinks, or hand grasps for "yes" and "no."
—Encourage communication despite the impairment; try guessing several possibilities; say "Do you mean . . . .?"
—In dealing with a dysphasic patient

- Speak slowly, use simple phrases, ask only one simple question at a time, repeat as needed.
- Allow plenty of time for the patient to answer questions.
- Do not treat the patient as if there is intellectual impairment (and thus instruct the family also); ask patient if he prefers for you to finish a sentence for him.
- Use gestures and other visual cues to add meaning to your words.

—Empathize with patient about how frustrating it must be not to be able to verbalize.
—Approach patient unhurriedly; talk directly to patient with sufficient light on you to enable patient to see your facial movements and body language.

—Phrase as many questions as possible so that patient can answer "yes" or "no."
—Teach patient with a tracheostomy to cover it while speaking; suggest a fenestrated trach tube.
—Consult speech therapist for speech rehabilitation program.
—Talk to patient; avoid talking only *about* the patient to others in presence of the patient.
—Establish a way the patient can call for help, such as a bell or a call light within reach; respond immediately to the call.
—Prepare families for possibility of labile emotions in the patient with a left hemispheric stroke; these patients become very frustrated and emotional when faced with their impaired speech.
—Be supportive, offer realistic encouragement; do not overestimate patient's language skills.

EVALUATION CRITERIA

The patient

—Uses some method of communication consistently.
—Demonstrates comprehension of spoken word.
—Begins to verbalize short phrases.

NURSING DIAGNOSIS

Impaired social interaction related to

—Cognitive impairment, memory deficits.
—Short attention span, confusion.
—Lack of motivation and/or of skills for social interaction.
—Difficulty in and/or inability to communicate.
—Decreased mobility.
—Depression.
—Emotional lability.

Social isolation related to

—Inability to participate in previous activities with friends or peers.
—Grief, depression.
—Fear of appearing in public with visible deficits.
—Inappropriate social behavior.
—Unwillingness of caregiver to be with patient in public.

GOALS

The patient will learn effective strategies for communicating; will maintain social interactions; will retain positive sense of self.

INTERVENTIONS

—Provide an accepting atmosphere; reduce environmental stress (for example, open curtains, decrease noise).
—Communicate empathy for the patient's problem; spend time with patient and show genuine interest.
—Encourage ventilation of feelings of frustration, fear, depression; indicate your understanding and acceptance.
—Explore strengths and resources that may help patient to socialize more comfortably; emphasize capabilities and reinforce sense of self-esteem.
—Inform patient that social withdrawl increases the sense of isolation and loneliness.
—Encourage visiting by significant others; keep family informed and involved in the patient's rehabilitation.
—Accept the patient's pattern of behavior and treat in a normal manner regardless of the level of response; the stimulation and sense of being included are important to recovery.
—Be alert to verbal and nonverbal cues indicating increased isolation, withdrawal, despair, suicidal ideation.

EVALUATION CRITERIA

The patient

—Expresses interests appropriate to age.
—Interacts with significant other(s).
—Maintains eye contact during conversation.
—Has no indication of hostility in voice or behavior.
—Is animated rather than sad.

CHAPTER 23

Sexuality-Reproductive Pattern

The sexuality-reproductive pattern involves the patient's perceived satisfaction or dissatisfaction with his or her own sexuality. Reproductive functions are also focused within this pattern. Neurologic impairments, particularly neuromuscular deficits, may interfere radically with the patient's sexual performance and therefore with the patient's perception of own sexuality.

The nursing diagnosis that is most useful for patients experiencing neurologic injury or dysfunction and associated with the sexuality/reproductive functional health pattern is sexual dysfunction.

Sexual Dysfunction. Sexual dysfunction may occur in many different populations of patients, but it may be more pronounced in patients with spinal cord injury. Loss of function, job, finances, friends, and significant others as well as physical isolation may contribute to sexual dysfunction either on a tempory basis or permanently.

NURSING DIAGNOSIS

Sexual dysfunction related to

—Lack of nerve innervation to genital area.
—Misinformation and lack of knowledge.

GOALS

The patient will understand the nature of the sexual dysfunction and options available within physical limitations; the patient and significant other will develop methods of sexual gratification and will participate in close interpersonal relationship.

INTERVENTIONS

—Wait until the patient is ready to assimilate information before taking the initiative to discuss sexual concerns and individual sexual functions and limitations; be sensitive to questions and needs.

—Inform patient that most people with spinal cord lesions can engage in some form of satisfying sexual activity, and that sexual abilities/limitations depend on the site of the lesion and degree of injury to the cord.

—Gather information about the patient's preinjury sexual functioning to determine realistic approaches to current sexual needs.

—Encourage patient to express feelings concerning sexuality, for example, loss of libido, and/or inability to have an erection, ejaculation, or orgasm.

—Offer information on sexual techniques using books, manuals, and movies as available.

—Emphasize the emotional aspects of sex, particularly if successful coitus is unlikely.

—Do not overrate importance of a physical sexual relationship to satisfactory lifestyle; nonphysical avenues of sexual expression can be satisfying.

—Encourage and assist the patient in maintaining personal appearance; wearing 'real' clothes and jewelry, using perfume, after-shave lotion.

—Foster and support the patient's tentative steps toward reestablishing intimacy with others.

—Foster open communication between patient and significant other.

—Act as the sounding board for family members to verbalize worries and concerns.

—Discourage inappropriate sexual flirtations by patient toward the nurse without undermining patient's self-confidence.

—Refer to expert counsellors when necessary." (Neal, Cohen and Reighley 1986: 112–113.)

—Provide for privacy if patient is allowed conjugal visits prior to discharge or during rehabilitation; encourage sexual exploration between patient and significant other to find new options not previously considered.

EVALUATION CRITERIA

The patient

—Maintains close relationship with significant other.
—Is well-groomed, neat, well-dressed.
—Asks questions about sexual functioning.
—Verbalizes an understanding of options available for sexual satisfaction.

SUGGESTED READINGS

Neal M, Cohen P, Reighley J: *Nursing Care Planning Guides. Set 6,* Baltimore, Williams & Wilkins, 1986.

CHAPTER 24

Coping-Stress Tolerance Pattern

The coping-stress tolerance pattern allows for the coordination of information regarding the patient's and family's coping abilities, stressors, and support systems. The challenges imposed on patients experiencing neurologic impairment and on their families may be excessive and the nurse needs to elicit information regarding coping and have ready access to a wide referral system.

The nursing disgnoses that are most useful for patients experiencing neurologic injury or dysfunction and associated with the functional health pattern of coping-stress tolerance, include ineffective family coping and ineffective individual coping.

Ineffective Family Coping. Sometimes the family suffers more pain than the patient after a family member is neurologically injured. The patient may not fully comprehend the impact of the injury on total family life. The patient may be able to provide little or no support to the rest of the family during the time they are making major changes. Prolonged disability may exhaust the supportive capacity of a family.

Ineffective Individual Coping. Everyone varies in the means with which stress is handled, whether it be a temporary stressor or a permanent one. Ineffective methods of coping with a situation increase energy consumption and prevent psychologic stability. Defense mechanisms that are used inappropriately fail to maintain psychologic equilibrium. Recognition of their inappropriateness can act as a guide to directing the patient and family toward appropriate use of defense mechanisms and other coping mechanisms.

NURSING DIAGNOSIS

Ineffective family coping related to

—Disruption of usual family life-style role changes.
—Burden of care.

—Hospitalization of family member.
—Changes in family member's appearance and/or role.

GOALS

The family will identify and use effective coping strategies to meet the challenges of caring for a chronically ill patient; will experience decreased anxiety.

INTERVENTIONS

—Make family aware that egocentricity and personality change is common, especially after head injury (for example, inappropriate social behavior, affect, hallucinations, delusions, altered sleep patterns).
—Evaluate the family's perception and repsonse to events necessitating patient's hsopitalization.
—Assess family's strengths and weaknesses with regard to their coping and problem-solving abilities; identify stressors to ineffective coping.
—Make referrals to community resources, such as support groups, social services for financial concerns for family.
—Urge primary caregivers to take time for themselves and to continue participation in outside interests; day-care centers and respite-care programs provide caregivers needed time away from the patient.
—Encourage family to use adaptive behaviors that have worked previously; suggest new options and coping behaviors that may be helpful.
—Support family through role adjustments (for example, the child is often put in the role of parent and vice versa when a patient is demented).
—Assist family and patient to form realistic expectations for performance of current and future roles.
—Encourage ventilation of feelings of guilt, anxiety, despair; provide empathy and show your understanding of the family's situation and responses.
—Give family information about patient's treatment and progress on a regular basis; encourage questions.
—Identify factors that may contribute to difficulty dealing with current situation; explore past experiences and support systems.
—Involve family in care of patient when possible.
—Discuss with family the underlying reasons for patient's behavior (for example, poststroke patient may use loud profanity even when the patient never used profanity before the stroke) to assist them to accept and support the patient during the illness.
—Show support and not disapproval if and when caregivers finally decide to institutionalize the patient with dementia.
—Educate family not to take it personally since it is often part of the illness

when a demented person accuses them of stealing or blames them unfairly.

—Instruct family to seek help regarding financial and legal issues (for example, obtaining power of attorney while the patient still has lucid intervals).

—Explain to family that early in dementia the patient may be stubborn, argumentative and use denial as a defense so that he does not have to acknowledge his declining intellectual function.

—Suggest to family that to avoid confusing a patient, the choices given to the patient may need to be limited (food eaten or clothes worn).

—Instruct the family to leave the area and call for help if the patient becomes combative to the degree that the caregiver's own safety is in jeopardy.

EVALUATION CRITERIA

The family

—Meet their own needs as well as those of the patient.
—Discuss personal problems, feelings, attitudes.
—Demonstrate effective and adaptive coping mechanisms
—Verbalize confidence to cope with the situation.

NURSING DIAGNOSIS

Ineffective individual coping related to

—Situational crisis.
—Inadequate and/or ineffective support system and/or coping mechanisms.
—Loss of control and independence.
—Inability to deal with severity of injury.
—Change in role and lifestyle, stress, irritability.
—Unrealistic perception of self or condition.
—Public stigma.

GOALS

The patient will effectively adapt to an altered appearance and abilities; will participate in care within limitations of illness; will develop positive ways to cope with illness.

INTERVENTIONS

—Review psychosocial history to help anticipate how the patient will comply with injury; knowledge of the patient's interest, hobbies, and leisure activities may assist the staff in stimulating the patient, especially during the phase of depression.

—Provide resources to family and patient regarding coping with the patient's deficits or disorder.

—"Provide an atmosphere of trust and caring to facilitate and encourage verbalization of patient's fears and concerns.

—Determine patient's ongoing strengths and values.

—Identify potential solutions to present problems and assist patient to set realistic goals.

—Assist [patient] to identify some new effective coping mechanisms; provide positive reinforcement when they are utilized.

—Encourage independence; problem solving promotes self-esteem.

—Encourage involvement of partner in coping process; this may assist patient to cope with stressors.

—Encourage active participation in self-care to maintain dignity and feelings of self-worth.

—Keep informed of physical condition to maintain or increase realistic perception of the diagnosis/prognosis.

—Explain disease process, diagnostic studies/treatments to help relieve anxiety or fear that may hinder the coping process.

—Refer to pastoral care as desired.

—Obtain social service and home care consults if necessary." (Caine R, Bufalino P: *Nursing Care Planning Guides for Adults.* Baltimore, Williams & Wilkins, 1987, p 377.) For example, patient may need help applying for Medicaid or Aid to Dependent Children, or may need support services such as Meals-on-Wheels.

—Offer support group participation if available.

—Assure that patient and family have accurate information about the situation and methods of handling potential problems that may arise.

—Assess family's effect on patient; allow more frequent visits if patient is more at ease with the family present; if patient seems more agitated or the ICP rises, minimize visits during the acute phase, explaining rationale to family.

EVALUATION CRITERIA

The patient

—Verbalizes feelings about the situation.

—Asks for help and support from others.

—Identifies individual strengths.

—Develops at least one new effective coping mechanism.

Index

Page numbers in *italics* denote figures; those followed by "t" denote tables.

normal, 20
normal physiology, 20–23
  cerebral perfusion pressure, 22–23
  compensatory mechanisms, 21
  Monro-Kellie doctrine, 20
  venous outflow, 23
  volume-pressure relationships, 21, 22
pathology, 23–28
waveform interpretation, 35, 36
Ismelin, for autonomic dysreflexia, 199
Isoproterenol, for vasospasm, 47

Jacksonian march, 74

Kaposi's sarcoma, 124
Kenny Self-Care Evaluation, 177
Kernig's sign, 68, 121
Kinesthetic stimulation, 171–172
Knowledge deficit, care plan, 219, 225–226
Kurtzke Status Scale, 177

Landry-Guillain-Barré syndrome. *See*
  Guillain-Barré syndrome
Landry's paralysis. *See* Guillain-Barré
  syndrome
Laser therapy, for spinal cord-injured
  patients, 101
Lasix. *See* Furosemide
Lecithin, for Alzheimer's disease, 152
Level of consciousness. *See also* specific states
  of consciousness
  alterations
    brain death, 23, 52, 55–56, 57t
    coma, 52–53, 54, 56, 58
    diagnosis, 58–59
    ethical issues, 59–63
    locked-in syndrome, 52, 55
    medical management, 59
    vegetative state, 52–55
  assessment, 3–5, 4, 5t
    abstract reasoning, 5
    Glasgow Coma Scale, 3–4, 5t
    orientation, 4–5
    recent memory, 5
    speech/language, 5
  definition, 51
  increased intracranial pressure and, 26
  reticular activating system and, 3, 4
  stages of anesthesia, 52–53
Lidocaine, for increased intracranial pressure,
  33

Lithium carbonate, for headache prevention,
  163
Living with Chronic Neurologic Disease, 178
Locked-in syndrome
  causes, 55
  classification, 55
  definition, 52
Low back pain, 163–166
  conservative therapy, 164
  diagnostic tests, 166
  etiology, 164
  incidence, 164
  surgical management, 164, 166
Lumbar puncture, 16–17
  cerebrospinal fluid examination, 16–17
  contraindications, 27
  headache and, 159, 162
  indications for, 16
  nursing intervention, 17
  for seizures, 78
  in subarachnoid hemorrhage, 45, 46
Luminal. *See* Phenobarbital
Lundberg waves, 35

Magnetic resonance imaging
  for increased intracranial pressure, 34
  nursing intervention, 19
Mannitol
  administration guidelines, 38
  for increased intracranial pressure, 29–30,
    140
Medulloblastoma, 108
Memory, 5
Meningioma, spinal, 116–117
Meningitis
  etiology/pathophysiology, 120–121
  management, 124–125
Meperidine, for headache, 162
Mephenytoin, for seizures, 80t
Mesantoin. *See* Mephenytoin
Mestinon. *See* Pyridostigmine bromide
Methotrexate, for brain tumor, 113
Methsuximide, for seizures, 81t
Methysergide, for headache, 159, 160t, 162
Metoclopramide, for nausea, 160
Metrifonate, for cysticercosis, 126
Midrin, for headache, 162
Migraine
  classic, 155–156
  common, 156
  complicated, 156
  treatment, 160t